A WEALTH OF EXPERIENCE

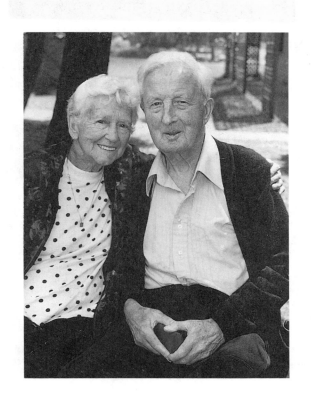

*This book is dedicated
to the memory of our Director*

TOM MACLENNAN
1943-1994

A WEALTH OF EXPERIENCE

A Guide to Activities for Older People

SECOND EDITION

MEREDITH BUDGE

Occupational Therapist
Carmel Hurst and Associates Consultancy Service, Melbourne

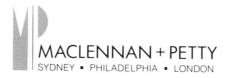

MACLENNAN + PETTY
SYDNEY • PHILADELPHIA • LONDON

First published 1989
Reprinted 1990
Second edition 1994

MacLennan & Petty Pty Limited
80 Reserve Road, Artarmon, NSW 2064, Australia

National Library of Australia
Cataloguing-in-Publication data:
Budge, Meredith
A wealth of experience
2nd ed.
Includes index
ISBN 0 86433 093 6
1. Aged – Australia – Recreation. 2. Occupational therapy for
the aged – Australia. I. Title
790.19260994

Printed and bound in Australia

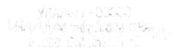

Contents

APPENDICES

Acknowledgements

There are many reasons why this book has come into existence, and many people to thank for their contributions, assistance and support.

Firstly, I'd like to thank the contributors to the book. They include Carmel Hurst, who is perhaps the inspiration behind most of the material in this book, as she was the inspiration behind South Port Community Nursing Home itself; Judy Stanton, who contributed to the sections on volunteers and students; the late Mary Jones, from Queen Elizabet Centre, Ballarat; Glenn Krusic-Golub of Grace McKellar House; Eunice Barter of Mayfield; Madge Williams of Sefton Lodge; Kay Waldron, who contributed material on visiting; Simone Keogh, the recreationist who also worked at South Port; Mary Ward, music therapist; Helen Scott, librarian from Council on the Ageing and Adriana Tiziana from the Alzheimer's Society.

In particular, I would like to thank Anne Smallpage, who took the photographs and provided all kinds of assistance with printing and selection.

There are many hidden contributors to this book. Barb Davison, occupational therapist and lecturer at Lincoln Institute, has been an invaluable source of advice and resource material. Robyn Twible reviewed and re-reviewed the work as it developed. Many community resource facilities freely offered information and help, particularly Jane Sharwood from the Victorian Department of Sport and Recreation. And all my working companions past and present, from Mt Royal Hospital, where the journey began, to all the different people from many different departments who have left their mark in one way or another. Jill Bothe and Cheryl Ellix were among the occupational therapists who have most fed my thoughts.

South Port Community Nursing Home — all its residents, staff and volunteers — are the authors of this work. Many of the residents, nurses, therapy, domestic and administrative staff, and volunteers came up with the ideas which are described here. I've just recorded them.

The continued support and input from Carmel Hurst and Associates has been essential to the development of the work. Carmel Hurst and Lyn Grocke have given much needed advice and support. They continue to remind me of the challenge and professional development which is available to anyone specialising in the geriatric field.

Another source of assistance has been Compuskill, a computer training program for unemployed people, which has helped to enter much of the data I have received from other contributors.

I thank the friends who have offered so much support in baby-minding, particularly Ros van Dalen and my mother (Mary Crook), Helen Tatai and Robyn Cocker.

And finally my husband, Tim, who offered valuable comments during the revision process and kept on believing in me and encouraging me throughout the entire hard slog.

Preface to the Second Edition

The last four years have seen a great deal of change in the aged care industry. The introduction of *Outcome Standards for Australian Nursing Homes* and the *Charter of Residents' Rights* have led to a marked improvement in the standards of care and quality of life for residents of many nursing homes and hostels. The emphasis on individual rights and freedom and on the need for a variety of experiences has meant that most nursing homes now employ activity workers. The Government Standards Monitoring Teams have placed particular emphasis on activity programs, even to the point where nursing homes risk closure if they do not give priority to activities.

The publication of the first edition of *A Wealth of Experience* was timely indeed, just as nursing home staff were seeking ways to meet the new standards. It has been exciting to be able to share in this process of change in the aged care industry.

It is now time for a revised edition. The first edition offered only limited activity ideas for the growing number of residents from other cultural backgrounds. This new edition helps us to explore ways in which we can cater for people of different nationalities, especially with our celebrations. This edition adds further information about collecting social histories, documenting activity programs and devising individual resident activity plans. It also includes other minor changes to broaden its scope for overseas markets, in the hope that we can share what we have learnt with aged care workers in other countries.

There is still much work to be done to improve and maintain the standard of care in every nursing home and hostel. We can never sit back and say, *at last we've done it*, because each new resident brings different needs and expectations to the aged care setting. So every activity program will be constantly changing and improving, to keep abreast with the needs of its clients.

Use this book well and you will join the growing number of staff in aged care centres who have discovered that activity programming is not only essential for quality of life, but also very rewarding and fun to provide.

Preface to the First Edition

South Port Community Nursing Home provided the venue, the staff, the residents and the volunteers through which to test most of the ideas presented in this book. Some creative program ideas from other settings are also included to provide a comprehensive reference for all workers in this field.

South Port is a community-based, deficit-funded, non-profit nursing home in Albert Park, Melbourne. It came into existence through the hard work and persistence of the local residents of South Melbourne and Port Melbourne. They saw the need and raised enough money to persuade the Federal Government to fund the rest of the project.

South Port belongs very much to the local community. Local residents have a very special commitment to the nursing home, and see it as another community facility which they have access to. Admission is based on need; the only other criterion is that applicants must either reside, or have key relatives or friends residing, in the prescribed Council areas. No one is excluded for financial reasons.

It houses 60 residents, 47 women and 13 men. Of these, 10% can walk with a stick for short distances only, while 90% require wheelchair transport. Many have had cerebrovascular accidents so have only unilateral upper limb function. More than 70% demonstrate some level of dementia. Many residents need assistance to participate in the activities, so volunteers and relatives play an important role in helping less able residents to take part.

Many of the ideas provided here may not be new, but at South Port Community Nursing Home they have worked exceptionally well. It is the level of participation by all staff, volunteers and the local community which makes these ideas work.

The book seeks to provide a model structure for an activities program and, at the same time, give easy access to the ideas and the recipes to make them work, in any setting. But remember, if you want your program

A WEALTH OF EXPERIENCE

to be more than a variety of bright moments in an otherwise dull week, look carefully at the whole structure of the facility and tackle it if you can.

I cannot stress sufficiently the fact that, in all these activities, 'people' resources are far more important than tools and equipment. The involvement of staff, relatives, friends and volunteers from the local community is essential. Other physical resources will automatically follow.

Author's note: Throughout this text a number of terms are used interchangeably; they can be read to mean their alternatives, depending on the setting to which this material is applied.

The terms 'resident', 'participant', 'person attending centre' and 'older person' are all used to describe those taking part in the organised programs. By design, the word 'patient' is not used, as these activities are geared towards encouraging people to assume active control over their lives. Patients are recipients of care.

'Nursing home', 'centre', 'aged care facility', 'hostel', 'special accommodation house' and 'extended care facility' are also interchangeable in most cases.

In addition, as most workers in the field and most older adults are female, I use 'she' and 'her' in preference to 'he' and 'him' in most cases, although the existence of men is recognised!

THE TOTAL APPROACH

Chapter 1
A Philosophical Framework

This resource manual is designed to help all those who provide activity and recreational programs for groups of older people in any setting within the community. It is directed particularly towards nursing home, special accommodation and hostel facilities, but it also provides valuable resource material for other community-based services, such as day hospitals, day centres, senior citizen groups, community centres, community socialisation clubs and voluntary agencies.

The book not only provides ideas and guidelines for the practical application of the various activities; it also presents a philosophical and structural framework within which to apply these ideas. The more theoretical and technical issues have not been addressed in this book because there are many other references already available which fulfil that role.

Activity programs for quality of life

The activity programs in this book seek to provide opportunities for residents to be involved in as many normal, fun, everyday activities as those who live in the wider community. It includes many familiar and regular activities such as gardening, cooking, woodwork, crafts and word games, as well as music, discussions and much reminiscing. Seasonal and calendar events supply themes to direct many of these activities.

There are parties and celebrations which involve the local community in the nursing home and provide a context for cooking and preparation activities as well as an opportunity to have fun. Outings occur regularly, both small and large.

More than anything else, the community will be actively involved in the life of the nursing home, just as residents will be actively involved in the community. Residents can attend community programs and go to local clubs. They may help to run a playgroup, or invite school groups to participate in their activities. Volunteers from the local community will come in to help or to run various group activities.

Such a program is designed to improve the quality of life of residents and to make sure that everyone — staff, friends, relatives and residents — enjoys themselves and wants to be involved in the lives of others.

What activity is not!

Let me dispel a few prejudices about activities for old people. To me, activity is many things. It is cuddling a baby, patting a dog, having a beer or getting ready for bed. It is having a shower, cooking a meal, visiting friends or just dozing in the sun. Activity, in this book, does not mean something you do in a craft room because Matron thinks it's 'good for you', or because there is an activity worker who needs to be kept busy. It is everything that you will do throughout the day which gives the day some sense of purpose and enjoyment, whether it is the pleasure of a long hot shower or going on an outing to the pub.

This may not be the dictionary meaning of 'activity', but it is certainly mine. It also means that everyone who happens to be in the building, for whatever reason, is a member of the team that provides the activity program.

A philosophical framework for activity programs

It is important to outline the basic premises which are essential to the application of quality of life programs. The next chapter gives a structural framework which will provide a base for the practical application of these philosophies. Subsequent chapters will describe the 'how to' or 'practice' required to make it all work.

PHILOSOPHY — STRUCTURE — PRACTICE

This is an important model for the provision of an activity program. If some of the activities described in this book are provided without the underlying principles presented in this model, they may actually work against the purposes of running quality of life programs.

What is the purpose of an activity program?

Let us stop to think for a moment of what it must be like for a person about to enter a nursing home. She must face the loss caused by some physical and/or mental disability which has forced her to give up home, family, pets and neighbours, in addition to her ability to exercise a free choice over her daily activities. She must enter a strange communal environment full of unfamiliar faces (which change constantly), confusing layout (Where on earth is the bathroom?) and a completely new life routine. It is difficult ever to understand fully the pain, loss and sense of displacement that each person entering an extended care facility must experience.

The centre must do all it can to reduce the stress of this great upheaval. A sensitive, patient, caring environment is needed to help each person adjust to this new lifestyle. A homelike environment, which offers positive opportunities for people to exercise choice and control over their lives, which encourages participation in pleasurable experiences, and which enables continued active involvement with friends and the local community will make this transition much easier.

So, the main purpose of running an activity program is to create an environment which offers the best possible quality of life for the residents of the centre. I must emphasise again that quality of life means that every person has the right to exercise active control and choice over every aspect of their lives. The environment must foster this.

A program designed to promote quality of life will also make sure that everyone has plenty of opportunities to have fun and laughter. This will be achieved by offering a variety of experiences and many chances for contact with other people.

The creation of a homelike environment which encourages individuals to take active control of their lives and participate in meaningful and enjoyable activities has one ultimate aim — to encourage the participants to maintain their dignity and self-esteem.

As we seek to fulfil this aim, we must always remember that we are workers in the home of a group of people. We must approach residents in a nursing home or hostel in the same manner as we would approach friends in their own home. We must respect each person's right to determine how they will live out their lives. Every staff member's role must include working to create a homelike environment, encouraging residents to see the centre as their home, not another hospital where all vestiges of self-determination are handed over to the staff 'who know best'.

Most people in these centres have lost some physical or mental capacity and thus are unable to actively control all aspects of their lives. It is therefore important that every remaining avenue through which to exercise control is made available. If not, the provision of activities may only become one more part of the institutionalised program which people attend because they are told it is good for them. Few people will gain quality of life from activities in which they feel forced to participate.

Why are these things important?

Everyone has the right to a fulfilling life, right until death. This is a well-documented human need. Older people who find themselves in special care, for whatever reason, are not exempt from this need for fulfilment; nor do they have any less right to it. Quality of life programs should aim to provide for fulfilment and a sense of well-being among the participants.

A loss of autonomy can lead to depression and withdrawal, and a greater degree of dependence in self-care.[1] This can only work against a sense of well-being and, therefore, real quality of life. It is no wonder that some residents maintain clear territorial divisions over their seating arrangements in the communal areas. Perhaps it is, for some, the last frontier of control over their lives.

It has been shown that socialisation and stimulation programs do more than improve the sense of well-being in residents. Significant improvements may occur in sleeping patterns, independence in self-care, and continence.[2,3] Some studies have shown that a lack of stimulation causes an increased rate of deterioration.[4]

Furthermore, after the age of 55, the nervous system becomes more vulnerable to sensory deprivation.[5] A person who is restricted to one location and has little opportunity for exercise and purposeful activity — in addition to the usual decreases in visual and hearing acuity in later years — is likely to suffer from significant deprivation. However, sensory stimulation programs can slow the deterioration process significantly and, as a result, encourage residents to maintain their independence, emotional stability and intellectual skills.[6]

So an activity program should seek to offer many chances for residents to use all their sensory abilities to the full. This is achieved by providing opportunity for movement, a variety of visual and auditory experiences, the chance to feel many different textures, to touch and be touched by others, and to experience a broad variety of tastes. Involvement in many normal activities will make this all possible.

In Australia nursing homes need to meet certain standards in order to remain in operation. The Federal Department of Community Services and Health has produced a document of Standards for Nursing Homes, which is the basis for requirements of all nursing homes throughout Australia.[7]

The standards include:

Objective 1. **Health care:** Residents' health will be maintained at the optimum level.

Objective 2. **Social independence:** Residents will be enabled to achieve the maximum degree of independence as members of society.

Objective 3. **Freedom of choice:** Each resident's right to exercise freedom of choice will be recognised and respected whenever this does not infringe upon the rights of other people.

Objective 4. **Homelike environment:** The design, furnishing and routines of the nursing home will resemble an individual's home as far as reasonably possible.

Objective 5. **Privacy and dignity:** The dignity and privacy of nursing home residents will be respected.

Objective 6. **Variety of experience:** Residents will be encouraged and enabled to participate in a wide variety of experiences appropriate to their interests and needs.

Objective 7. **Safety:** The nursing home environment and practices will ensure the safety of residents, visitors and staff.

These objectives are described in full in the document. The details of these requirements clearly support the need for comprehensive quality of life programs for residents in these centres. The objectives demonstrate future federal policy directive and can be strong arguments for change in our extended care facilities. Use them well to support the introduction of new activities and programs.

What an activity program cannot do without

The following requirements are the essential elements of the philosophical framework so far described.

Choice

As already stated, in order to foster quality of life, the environment must offer residents the opportunity to exercise control over all aspects of their lives: over the nature of their surroundings, the type and extent of their medical care, the time they get up, what and how much they eat, their use of tobacco and alcohol (while not imposing on others), what they wear, the activities they choose to participate in, and the people they meet.

To meet the varied interests of residents, a wide range of choices must be provided but the facility must also provide the option for residents to decline involvement in activities.

Homelike environment

The physical environment of the centre should be as homelike as possible. Although every nursing home and special accommodation home will not be new or purpose-built, it is possible to ensure that the environment is warm, well lit and comfortable. Heating and cooling should be adequate. It may be necessary to replace some windows and install skylights, for example, to introduce as much natural lighting as possible. Furnishings should be safe and comfortable and yet, at the same time, homelike rather than sterile and purely functional.

The environment will be further enhanced if residents are encouraged to surround themselves with their own belongings and furniture. It can make a tremendous difference to see one's own chest of drawers, favourite chair and footstool in use instead of hospital furnishings.

However, furnishings are not enough. A family atmosphere is essential to the creation of a homelike environment. In my experience, the friendship and familiarity between staff and residents and their families contributes more to the residents' sense of mental well-being than, for example, a structured reality orientation program. All staff should be encouraged to contribute significantly to the lives of the residents, not just those who are professionally involved. For example, the domestic staff can often form the most lasting friendships because of their regular shifts and low changeover rates. Their involvement in outings and activities is therefore most worthwhile. The hairdresser is another person who plays a significant role in the lives of residents.

It is also important to be aware of each individual's preference for companionship. As people get to know each other, bonds can develop between those who have most in common with each other or have compatible personalities. This is a very normal process which should be respected, and one which can contribute significantly to the creation of a family atmosphere.

The careful selection of staff and continued education through an in-service program play a very important role in creating and maintaining a family atmosphere and therefore a normal homelike environment.

Most people in the community keep pets or have some contact with animals so a normal home environment will probably include pets. A dog, cat and budgie should be in residence at every facility. Relatives, staff and volunteers can also be encouraged to bring in their pets regularly.

Community involvement

Providing a program geared towards enhancing quality of life means, in particular, including opportunities for residents to be involved in the lives of other people. Community involvement is an essential part of quality of life programs and residents should have many opportunities to join with others in the local community. There is a great resource of activities in the community which residents can take part in and, if used to the full, they can reduce the strain on the nursing home's own resources. Residents can attend community art, recreation and education programs. They can go to local clubs and neighbourhood groups. They may be able to offer tutorship programs for school students, or creche assistance, or help run a playgroup. Many guest performers and talented volunteers from the local community will come in to offer entertainment or run various activity groups.

Activities

The program should base its approach on the important principle of participation in normal, familiar activities. Such activities help to identify one day from the next and provide landmarks throughout the year. In so doing, the program stimulates interest in life generally.

Purposeful activity

There must be a focus or purpose for involvement in activities. Activity for its own sake alone does not contribute to a sense of worth in those taking part. The emphasis will be to encourage participants to feel useful and able to contribute significantly to the lives of others.

So, activities are geared towards events which occur throughout the calendar year. Crafts are made for gifts or fundraising. Food is cooked for parties and for eating! The garden club is directed towards the centre's own garden needs. Games are played with children or for social contact. Yet, in everything, having fun is just as much a justification for an activity. Hence, parties are also a big part of the program.

Reminiscing

The chosen activities will also need to offer chances for people to share their past memories, for reminiscing is an important part of the older person's life. The need to think through and discuss past events is not necessarily evidence of short-term memory loss, but can be a normal process stemming from a person's need to review her life as she approaches death. The program should seek to accommodate this need, and staff should be encouraged to spend time chatting and listening. Activities can centre upon events from people's pasts; this may evoke old memories and encourage participants to discuss them. An important tool for this is described in Chapter 14 — a photo album which records photographs and memories of a person's life will contribute immensely to a person's ability to reflect upon their past.

In summary

If all these principles and guidelines are followed, then the activity program that grows from this base will offer its participants the opportunity to improve significantly their sense of well-being and quality of life.

The cultural population

Recognising the culture of the centre

No aged care facility will house people of entirely the same culture or background, and it is important to be aware of the different personalities and cultural backgrounds of the residents before launching an activity program. The area in which the home is situated, the educational and employment histories of the residents, and the life experiences of each individual will influence the degree of interest shown in the various activities. Careful assessment of these factors will help to ensure that the program matches the interests of the participants.

An example of one cultural setting

For example, some of the ideas presented in this book were introduced in an area where many of the people were used to hard work rather than leisure and craft activities. A few drinks, card games and plenty of jokes leaning over the public bar were the common practice. As a result, this group was generally not interested in crafts and had limited enthusiasm for educational programs, but enjoyed parties with singalongs and plenty of socialising.

Of course, a significant number of residents did not match this general description and their needs and interests were catered for within smaller group and individual activities. There was a special classical music group; some worked on individual craft projects while others attended classes outside the home, either at the local high school with school students or through the 'Learning for the Less Mobile' program. Outings varied in venue and group size to cater for the different interests of residents.

Staff are all encouraged to respond to the specific interests of individuals. For example, a shared interest in racing may lead to a staff member taking a resident to the races, or another staff member may take a resident to the Easter Passion play at her church.

Multicultural backgrounds

Many centres will house people whose cultural backgrounds originate from completely different countries. This will create an even greater variance in the style of life these people are used to. As stated in the standards document, *Living in a Nursing Home*[7], a person's right to exercise cultural practices must be respected. Multiculturalism must be recognised and integrated into the life of our aged care facilities. People from various nationalities bring a wealth of experiences and interests which can contribute significantly to the life of the home. The celebration of national events and the introduction of music, food and activities from different cultures is just the beginning of this necessary process.

Religious preferences

Religious preferences should be observed. Mass, a church service or other religious activities can be held at the centre. If the resident wishes, family members or friends should be encouraged to take their relative to their local church or religious centre.

A passive lifestyle

The lifestyles of people will vary in other ways, too. Some will prefer an active life, others a far more passive one. There will be some residents who are not interested in any activities. Some people feel they have worked hard all their lives and deserve a rest. It is very important to respect these

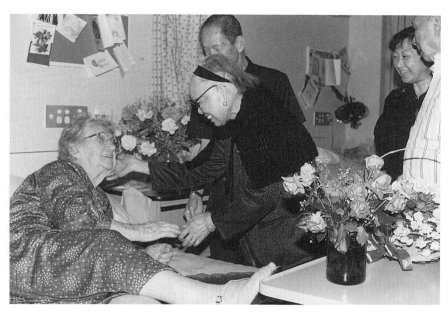

Visitors from the local Chinese community greet residents for Chinese New Year.

wishes. The right, and opportunity, to say no is perhaps more important than actually being involved in an activity. Beware of other staff members who feel certain residents miss out because they choose not to be involved. There can be hidden pressure to get people to join in, although it is against their will. However, by getting to know the resident well, this can be avoided.

Good and bad days

Recognise the varying moods of each person. There will be many 'off' days when a normally active resident will simply feel like being alone and quiet for the day. Respect the wishes of residents even if it seems they are going to miss a great opportunity. If the organiser or other staff member knows the resident well enough, they will learn when to encourage and when to leave the person in peace.

In summary

In each different setting the needs and interests of the residents will vary greatly, and not all the ideas presented in this book will be appropriate. Some activities can be adapted to suit the population, but it is very important to get to know residents and their interests before introducing too many new ideas. (See the Socialisation Assessment form in Chapter 17, p. 242.)

Influencing the culture of the centre

Changes take time

Talking with people and listening to them is the best way to plan appropriate activities. However, it is important not to limit the program only to those activities which the resident has already experienced. Many may not be aware of the options available to them and will find they unexpectedly enjoy new activities. It is a good idea to try a new event and then ask the residents for feedback.

Many of the activities need to be introduced gradually. Don't expect people who are used to sitting in rows, with little to do all day, suddenly to jump at the chance to join in a major activity. Introduce changes in the structure of the home before tackling too many activities. Start small, and build from there. For example, test the sense of humour of residents by wearing a crazy hat and watch for the reaction before introducing special events with costumes.

Encouraging participation

Participation is encouraged by placing activities in a central location, such as the lounge, so that residents can observe the fun and decide if they would also like to participate. By presenting most of the activities in the main lounge area, many residents who do not actually want to take part can at least enjoy the atmosphere, join in the conversation and have a few laughs with the participants.

But the need for uninterested residents to withdraw must also be respected and the home should provide a number of quiet areas where residents can enjoy peace. In addition, some of the activities will require a quiet environment, free from distractions. Residents should be consulted to ensure they are happy for their lounge to be used in this fashion.

Although many residents like to participate in an activity, they often do not want to move too far from their usual spot for fear of missing visitors. Activities which do take people out of the home or to another room need plenty of prior warning, so that arrangements can be made with relatives and friends. If the activity room is just off the main living area, this becomes less of a problem.

By introducing activities in this manner, with constant review from the residents' committee, the atmosphere of the home can be developed and changed over time, to improve the quality of life of the residents.

Conclusion

Organisers of activity programs must always keep in mind the purpose of the program. It is not there just to make life exciting, but to ensure that each individual within the centre can exercise choice and control over his or her life, and thus enhance its quality. To foster this quality of life, a homelike environment is needed, both in appearance and atmosphere. There is also a need for the residents to be involved in the local community, and in a selection of activities which interest them. Finally, if the cultural diversity of residents is recognised and respected, an activity program can be developed and introduced with sensitivity. You can then be sure that the program really will work to improve the quality of life of its participants.

References

1. Shultz R, Aderman D. Clinical research and the stages of dying. *Omega, Journal of Death and Dying.* 1974; 5:137–143.
2. Butler RN, Lewis MI. *Aging and Mental Health: positive psychological and bio-medical approaches.* CV Mosby, 1982; 336, 378–380.
3. Allen J. The use of isometric exercises in a geriatric treatment program. *Geriatrics.* 1965; 20:346–347.
4. Parent LH. Effects of low stimulus environments on behaviour. *American Journal of Occupational Therapy.* 1978; 32(1):19–25.
5. Lipowski ZJ. Delirium, clouding of consciousness and confusion. *Journal of Nervous Mental Disorder.* 1967; 145:225–227.
6. Bower HM. Sensory stimulation and the treatment of senile dementia. *Medical Journal of Australia.* 1967; 1(22):1113–1119.
7. Commonwealth/State Working Party on Nursing Home Standards: *Living in a Nursing Home. Outcome Standards for Australian Nursing Homes.* Australian Government Publishing Service, Canberra, 1987. Used with permission from AGPS. Copies of the report can be obtained from Commonwealth Government bookshops in Canberra and all State capitals or by Mail Order Sales, Australian Government Publishing Services, GPO Box 8, Canberra, ACT 2601.

Chapter 2

A Structural Framework

A structural framework is required to make sure the philosophies described so far are applied and maintained, and to provide a base for the practical application of the activity programs. This chapter will look at the people, processes and resources which are essential to the program's application. No amount of creative activities will fully meet the needs and interests of residents, and ensure quality of life, if these structures are not established.

One model of a staff structure

To demonstrate the ideal staff requirements and services for a successful program, I will describe the situation in which most of the ideas in this book were tested. It will provide a comparative model for other centres of varying size, facilities and cultural background, and can be adapted to meet the needs of each centre.

These programs were run in a 60-bed nursing home by an occupational therapist working 25 hours a week, in conjunction with a coordinator of volunteers working 12 hours and a physiotherapist working 20 hours. In addition to these permanent staff, other department members contributed to the program as they were able.

The nursing department contributed significantly to all activities by the way they prepared the residents for the day, by suggesting ideas, and by planning and participating in the subsequent activities. Domestic and reception staff offered a special source of stable long-term friendship and involvement. A large resource of people power was also available through the involvement of volunteers, relatives and community groups.

It helps if centre managers support such involvement of staff in the activity program. The increase in staff morale more than compensates for any time lost doing normal work. I have found that people generally work more efficiently in a fulfilling environment.

Although I am an occupational therapist, the position of activity co-ordinator could also be filled by someone with recreation qualifications or diversional therapy training. The coordinator of volunteers can likewise come from a variety of professional backgrounds. Personality and relevant experience contribute significantly to the selection of such staff. An occupational therapist may act as a consultant to ensure the activities match the abilities of the participants. The issues of assessment and consultancy will be discussed in a later chapter.

The involvement of all staff in this way means an inherent team structure is developed which ensures that the program will continue along similar lines, even during those inevitable gaps which occur between one activity coordinator's departure and the employment of the next.

Essentials of a structural framework

The following committees and service provision are necessary to ensure that an activity program really does respond to the needs and interests of residents.

Residents' committee

This meets once a month, organised by a staff member, such as the activity worker or coordinator of volunteers. All alert residents are encouraged to attend. Where possible, the residents assume roles of chairperson and secretary. Before the meeting, the chairperson and staff member develop the agenda together. Other staff attend upon invitation only.

The committee provides a forum for residents to discuss the continuing program, to consider new projects, air complaints about any aspect of life at the home, and to make recommendations about facilities, diet, activities, and so on. The meeting also delegates residents to write letters of thanks to various people/groups who contribute to the program. These could be dictated to a volunteer.

The residents' committee is essential in planning a program which meets the interests of the residents themselves. It enhances a sense of control and autonomy among residents.

Program committee

This meets once a month, usually convened by the activity coordinator. The coordinator of volunteers and a representative from each department, including therapy staff, nursing, domestic, kitchen and administration, attend this meeting. Regular commitments are noted, then activity and party ideas are suggested. A brainstorming session follows to plan celebratory days and outings usually with exciting and innovative results. The meeting also ensures that all departments are aware of the coming events and the likely demands these will place on their resources.

A large yearly planner calendar enables the activity organisers to maintain a thorough overview of the range and regularity of activities and events. They then can quickly assess if the program is really meeting the needs and requests of the participants.

Advertising

A weekly program sheet should be displayed around the building to inform everyone of the week's activities. A whiteboard in the lounge is useful for advertising the daily program. Special events which are coming up in the near future can be advertised with posters. This advance notice is important. Older people often prefer structure and stability in their lives, and need plenty of warning about coming events in order to prepare themselves for them. Advertising also ensures that everyone is aware of the choices available to them over the coming weeks.

In-service training

In-service educational sessions lasting about 45 minutes should, ideally, occur each week. Outside speakers are often invited to talk about their specialty areas. Internal staff can also run many of the sessions. Topics range from procedural techniques to social issues which affect everyone in the community. All staff are invited to participate. This process enables staff to understand the philosophy and practice required to maintain a high standard of care and quality of life for residents.

Support for relatives

It is important to offer support to relatives of new residents as they adjust to the new situation of their family member. It can be as difficult for families to adjust to the placement of their relative in residential care as it is for the person being placed. Feelings of loss, guilt, loneliness and uselessness are not uncommon. A social worker may be employed for a number of hours to work with the relatives, through support groups and counselling. The visiting program described in Chapter 13 also addresses this issue.

People: our best resource

People resources are far more important than tools and equipment and the involvement of staff, relatives, friends and volunteers from the local community is essential. Physical resources will automatically follow. Below is an outline of the roles various personnel can play in the life of the centre.

Relatives

Relatives are encouraged to participate and/or assist wherever they feel able — in regular groups, outings, vacations or parties. Relatives are particularly helpful in encouraging less able residents to take part in the program. They can lend an extra hand, provide one-to-one supervision where it is needed, or just add immensely to the social atmosphere of the

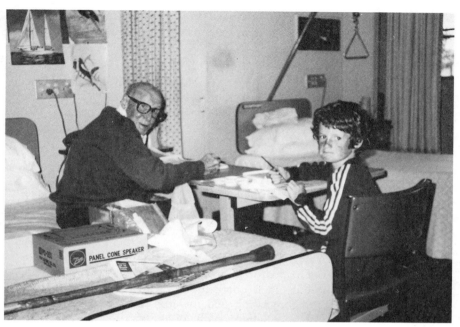

A nurse's child joins a resident to do some painting.

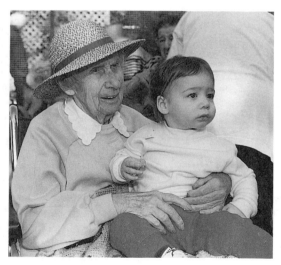

A doting great-grandmother looks forward to visits from her great-granddaughter.

group. Some relatives, however, will need direction from the group leader
to ensure that they assist rather than take over the role of the participant.

Children

Grandchildren and great-grandchildren, children of staff and volunteers
are all welcome to participate in activities with residents. Babies are a
must! The most confused person will respond appropriately, and with
great pleasure, to a baby; and everyone else just loves the chance for a
cuddle and a chat.

Schools

School teachers and children provide a wonderful resource for many activities. Community liaison teachers are particularly good resource people.

Volunteers

The opportunities for involvement are as wide as the interests of the
volunteers themselves. The coordinator of volunteers assesses each volunteer's interests and abilities, and channels them into appropriate areas.
Tasks include distributing morning tea, making beds, running groups,
providing entertainment and helping with all the various activities and
events. Volunteers of all ages can contribute and many move into new
areas of activity as their confidence develops (see Chapter 10).

Other staff

Use the individual talents of staff. This may mean encouraging a domestic
staff member's talent for making decorations, or for music, while tapping
into another's interest in racing. Musical ability, hobbies and interests
should be made use of wherever possible. Domestic and administrative
staff often work more predictable shifts than other staff and so are particularly able to develop lasting friendships with residents. This should be
encouraged.

Management committee

There is no better way of gaining support for creative programs than to
involve members of the management committee or other administrative
bodies in the fun. They can help in the planning of some events, receive
invitations to attend parties, and even join outings and vacations if they
wish. As a result, a healthy relationship will develop between management
and other staff and residents. The management will gain a more accurate
view of the benefits of the program, and thus offer greater support and
encouragement. Their involvement will also help to break down any
unhealthy barriers of hierarchy, which tend to stifle an atmosphere of
participation, teamwork and fun.

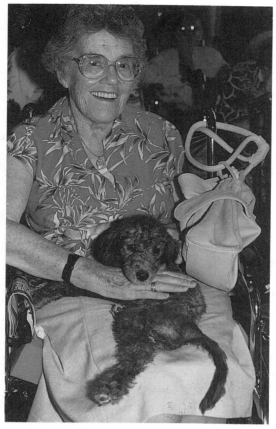

*Dogs are always popular whether the in-house
pet or a visitor.*

Pets

Animals are also very important in contributing to a sense of quality of life. Many older people have lived with pets all their lives. Pets provide a companionship and touch that humans cannot replace. A dog, cat, budgies, fish should all be part of the life of any aged care facility. It is important to find sociable animals which will share their affection around an entire home. Dogs, particularly, also offer residents an important sense of security.

Staff requirements: the essentials

Some of the activities described can be simplified so that anyone can run them. Others will require experienced and qualified staff to ensure their success. Without the staff described earlier in the chapter, the program will be limited in size and in frequency of events and activities, yet a lively atmosphere and a range of activities and madcap moments can exist with limited resources. Careful selection of staff and the content of the in-service programs will help to influence the atmosphere of the centre. Consultants can be called upon to oversee programs or make recommendations about the program development where necessary.

Job description

In order to be an effective member of a team, it is important that the worker and her colleagues have a clear idea of their roles and others' expectations of them. Each position needs to be recognised and valued. Too often I have seen the efforts of good activity workers undermined by the need to perform nursing duties from 8–10am, before struggling on to find the energy to run activities for the remainder of the day. Morning nursing is exhausting work and activity provision requires much energy, patience and resourcefulness. One of the most effective ways to improve an activity program is to give the activity worker permission to concentrate her efforts on activities provision. A job description is therefore essential. A sample job description is included at the end of this chapter. The activity worker should then have the opportunity to review and adapt the job description with management.

Employment initiatives

It is not within the scope of this book to discuss local employment initiatives but, just as we need to respond creatively to the development of activities, we also need to look creatively at ways of providing the people needed to operate effectively. If money is not available for a required position, we need to look to other sources such as trusts, employment programs, fundraising, sponsorship or self-funding programs. Chapters 9 and 10 give further information on community resources and volunteers.

Physical resources: the essentials

Facilities

The area where activities occur should be bright and attractive, with good lighting and plenty of windows. It should be close to the main living areas and accessible to independent wheelchair users. An extensive storage area is also necessary, preferably of the walk-in type, which allows a wide range of materials to be stored in an organised manner.

Equipment

This list is by no means exhaustive but it will provide a basic guide for those starting from scratch.

Tools

- tables
- chairs with arms
- blackboard
- scissors
- stationery items
- gardening tools
- woodwork handtools
- cooking utensils, including one-handed aids
- storage containers
- 'Stable Tables' (useful for individual work)
- library of craft, cooking, quiz and folklore books
- small oven/cook top
- carpet bowls
- skittles/quoits
- range of board games

Access to kitchen supplies and equipment may be necessary if there is not a kitchenette close to the activity area. Access to maintenance department tools is also helpful.

Music   A portable stereo system which has radio, cassette, and compact disc player in the one unit is most useful. Participants are then not restricted to a limited area to listen to music.

Outings   Access to a wheelchair bus is essential (see Chapter 9 for resource possibilities).

Audiovisual   Access to a 16mm projector and screen, and a slide projector, is also useful. These can often be borrowed from the local library or school.

Consumable resources

This is just the beginning of a list of basic consumable requirements.

Materials

- paints, brushes, pencils, textas, chalk
- glue, paper, cardboard, crêpe paper
- streamers, balloons
- old hats, ribbons, scraps of material, sewing materials
- novelty collections (for costumes)
- soil, seeds, seedlings, garden pots

- woodwork materials, wood, sandpaper, paint
- cooking ingredients other than kitchen supplies

The bar Throughout our lives, we all have the freedom to decide on our consumption of alcohol, and older people should also have the freedom to control this aspect of their lives. One way of meeting this need is to provide a bar. This should be situated in the lounge, with a fridge and storage space for beer, sherry, wine and soft drinks. Use light beer in preference to the heavier beers. The cost of the drinks can be shared by those residents who partake. Pre-lunch drinks can be served daily.

On party days extra supplies are ordered, and the bar remains open for longer periods. Some fundraising may be necessary to cover the cost of extra supplies. Your local liquor store may often be prepared to make special donations for these events. Staff and guests are invited to bring drinks to share.

Tobacco As smoking can be one of the few pleasures left for some older people, it is perhaps unfair to restrict its use, except where supervision is required for safety reasons. But non-smokers also have the right to smoke-free areas. A smoking room may need to be set aside, supervised by staff who also smoke. Alternatively, residents who wish to smoke may need to be rugged up and taken outside for their regular puff. This is an uncomfortable solution but one which is least likely to cause risk to the

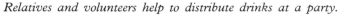
Relatives and volunteers help to distribute drinks at a party.

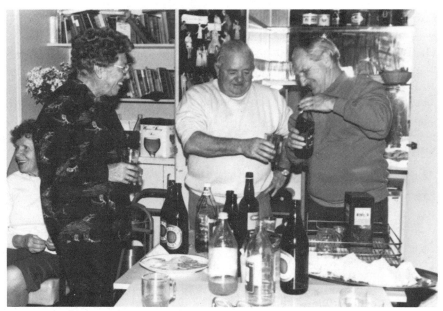

health of others, especially staff members. The residents' committee is the best forum to discuss these issues.

Finance Limited therapy department budgetary funds are used for the program, where necessary, although most activities cost little. We ran our program one year on a joint occupational therapy/physiotherapy annual budget of $500. (However, this certainly should not be considered adequate — it has since been increased!) The activity worker must have an annual budget allocated to them, with which to plan adequately for events and activities. Some fundraising through the sale of jams and crafts is also useful. Where possible, kitchen supplies fund all cooking activities. On celebratory days, staff and guests are often asked to contribute food and drink to share (see Chapter 3 for further fundchasing ideas).

Conclusion

With committees and meetings in place, and a strong commitment to involving everyone — residents, all staff, relatives, friends, volunteers and animals — in the life of the home at every level, the centre will be well on the way to providing comprehensive quality of life programs for its residents. If this kind of involvement does occur, the program will become far more varied and creative and, as a result, everyone will enjoy themselves in some way.

Sample job description for activity worker

Job title and qualifications:

The Activity Officer can hold a Diversional Therapy qualification, Red Cross certificate, Allied Health Assistant Certificate or have gained relevant work experience in the fields of aged care and/or activity.

Responsible to:

Director of Nursing, and initially, consultant Occupational Therapist.

Purpose:

The Activity Officer will work with other staff to promote the quality of life of the residents of the nursing home.

Tasks and responsibilities:

1. Plan the activity program in association with the Program Committee comprising representatives from nursing and domestic staff, residents and interested relatives.

   The program may include: celebratory days, musical activities, outings, special dinners, group and individual activities, contact with relatives and friends, involvement of children, school groups and community groups, and other activities requested by residents and staff.

2. With the assistance of other staff, coordinate and implement the program.

3. Provide weekly and monthly programs which will be displayed for staff, relatives and residents to refer to.

4. Encourage residents to participate in the planning of activities. Assist the resident and relatives committee to meet regularly.

5. In addition to the abovementioned activities, work towards involving residents in as many everyday, normal activities as would naturally occur in a home environment, including gardening, cooking, sweeping, folding clothes, singing, socialising and exercise.

6. Through discussion with residents, other staff and relatives, develop a good knowledge of the interests and abilities of residents.

7. Review social histories and develop individual activity plans for each resident, with the assistance of the Director of Nursing, other staff and relatives.

8. Keep statistics of activity participation and provide limited documentation as recommended.

9. Encourage and contribute to the creation of a more homelike physical environment within and surrounding the home.

10. Establish storage and activity areas within the home.

11. Administer any funds made available for activities through a petty cash system.

12. Attend support groups for workers in aged care, and/or seminars which will provide ongoing education, peer support and information resources.

13. Other tasks as they arise which are appropriate to the position and skills of the person appointed. The Activity Officer will not be required to perform nursing or domestic duties, other than those which relate directly to the provision of activities, for example, helping a resident to sweep, garden or cook.

Chapter 3

The Involvement of other Professionals

Part 1: The Place of Nursing in an Activities Program

*by Carmel Hurst**

The delights of working with old people in any care situation are unexpected, and probably not very obvious to the outsider. At a time when the roles of all those working in this area and their relationships to each other are being redefined, the importance of the nurse's role in aged care cannot be over-estimated.

As a nurse, I feel that the new emphasis being placed on the non-medical model, on freedom and anti-institutionalisation, is a wonderful chance for us all to get off on a new footing together. We can now begin to use new and imaginative techniques in caring for old people and promoting well-being, self-care and independence.

Our new approaches are based on the realisation that the needs of the individual throughout life are dynamic; the capacity to fulfil them alters with the biological as well as the psychosocial manifestations of ageing. More simply, we do not change in the things we need and like, but ageing modifies opportunity, refines tastes and often affects our ability to get what we want. Some things are easier, others are harder.

I believe our responsibilities as carers have much to do with providing background assistance to those who experience a gap between need and fulfilment. We have no place in a situation where there is no gap, except to offer community education if it is wanted.

An attractive vehicle to describe the role of activities for older people is Havinghurst's 'developmental tasks of later maturity'.[1] They help to clarify the areas where a person may be experiencing such a gap. They are:

---

* Carmel Hurst was the director of nursing at South Port Community Nursing Home in its developing years and the driving force behind its success as a leading centre in aged care. She has wide experience in geriatric nursing, and now runs Carmel Hurst & Associates, a consultancy service for workers in aged care.

25

- adjusting to declining physical strength and health
- adjusting to retirement and reduced income
- adjusting to death and bereavement
- establishing an explicit affiliation to one's own age group
- adopting and adapting social roles in a flexible way
- establishing satisfactory living arrangements

A quick look at this model suggests that our traditional way of doing things was not likely to further the welfare of an individual trying to make these kinds of adjustments. For instance, in the case of institutional care, you will remember the 'OT palace' in the hospital grounds, to which the patients were delivered, clean, dressed and toileted, for whatever it was that happened there. This occurred a maximum of three times a week and depended heavily on school holidays and the availability of porters. The traditional model certainly did not address such issues as death and bereavement, social adaptation and a satisfying lifestyle.

Instead, the traditional approach has led to other things. Interdisciplinary jealousies and lack of understanding have flourished under this system. Confusion over goals and methods have caused dissatisfaction for consumers, workers and policy makers.

The new way of thinking about our roles is much easier for me to understand and gives me more satisfaction. As nurses, it means that we do not have to limit ourselves to physical tasks with traditionally poor cultural value. It calls for lots of role-blurring, cooperation, understanding and mutual respect for the workers, client group and the family involved.

The new model means that everyone is involved together in helping residents participate in activities. Yet 'activities' itself has become a difficult word to deal with, as it has been over-used and now has stylised meanings for many people. For some it means therapeutic discussion groups, for others it means knitting infinite numbers of coat-hanger covers in the craft room on Wednesday afternoons.

I am concerned with helping nurses and others to realise the value of the activities they undertake, which can be mundane but should be meaningful. Preparing for a party or outing or just dressing to meet friends is the solid stuff of life. The discussion about choice of soap, perfume, jewellery and clothes, the conversations with friends in anticipation of an event, the planning for it, the involvement in it and the post-mortem after it, are all part of a complete cycle.

Just as there is little point in getting up and dressing in the morning if the day is only spent waiting for the night, so there is little meaning in being involved in activities if one is not well-groomed, comfortable and spiritually prepared.

Nursing priorities

Nursing is a curious business. It is a profession that nurses have a great deal of difficulty in defining. However, it has much to do with supplementing the needs of the individual when a gap occurs between need and the ability to fulfil it. This definition covers a lot of ground and has an omnibus element as well as a definitive one which is ours alone. Nurses are responsible for seeing that the basic survival indicators are there: food, clothing, shelter, elimination, cleanliness, etc.

Therefore, they are ultimately responsible for seeing that the person is clean, dry, well-dressed and rested in preparation for the day's events. At the same time, nurses perform a coordinating role by ensuring that activities are timed, safe and known about.

'Activities' happen all day long and in my mind I equate the word with everything a person needs to nourish the spirit: touch, conversation, laughter, bargaining, thinking and feeling. These activities meet all our non-physical needs, including the need for sensory stimulation and chances to use our cognitive abilities. This meaning insists that nurses are involved heavily at all times. Or, to put it another way, traditional nursing activities should contain these elements. A cuddle and a cup of tea are, perhaps, the best sleeping draught, and this nursing procedure might be described as an activity.

Nurses need reassurance that they will not be burdened with a pleasant social activity as an accustomed chore rather than as a spontaneous break from their usual work. The physical care of old people with extensive dependencies is demanding, and I know that many nurses deliberately avoid social interaction with residents for this reason. Nurses may need help to discard some tasks which prevent them from finding time to develop deeper friendships with those in their care.

When there is a party, for example, all staff should do the bare minimum of their normal work so they can participate to the full in the day's events. The beds could be left till after lunch and there is certainly no point in letting the cleaners do too much work before or during a party. There will be plenty to do later!

I think it is fair to say that many of us who are caring for old people have been trained in the acute medical model. This makes it very hard for us to adjust our thinking to the needs of people in extended care situations, people with different priorities. Because a new approach is now being taken, workers for whom this is news do not need to be criticised. They need to be supported and understood as they seek to adjust to the changes which they are being asked to implement.

Nurses will have to identify for themselves the relevance of time-honoured traditions, the validity of the priorities set for them, the limitations of the nursing role and their responsibility for self-assertion. There is need for improvement, but this is so for all professional disciplines. Perhaps the occupational therapist committed to the endless production of nylon bath mats could help the nurse with a fetish for tidiness and ruling lines in exercise books.

One has to accept that professionals who perform ritualistic activities have fears about the components of their work. The challenge, then, for those involved in developing an activities program is to seek to present new ideas in such a way as to lower this fear level as far as possible. This is necessary in order to obtain maximum cooperation, if not to counter downright obstructionism.

The team

Inter-professional rivalries are ridiculous. Our place in the team should not depend upon our notions of the relevance of our education to a professional pecking order, but upon the needs of the client. In my last place of work, two of the best activity officers we had were the receptionist and the laundry lady. We are all important. We are interdependent. There is plenty of original, creative work for each of us to do.

Historical context

The historical context in which extended care facilities have developed in our culture is not helpful to our present care needs. Many buildings now used to house our old people were once charity-supported almshouses. They were sponsored by individuals and societies who used such expressions as:

'. . . charitable relief to diseased, infirm, incurable, poor or destitute persons'.[2]

I feel sure that the physical surroundings in which some of us are living or working inspire traditions which are not consistent with freedom, self-determination and risk-taking. Refuges of this sort were probably never much fun.

Humour

This brings me to the subject of humour.

'Humour is a serious business. It can serve as a powerful tool for leaders at all levels to prevent the build-up of stress, to improve communication, to enhance motivation and morale, to build relationships, to encourage creative problem solving . . .'[3]

There is nothing solemn about old or disabled people that puts them outside the general need that we all have for fun and humour. Norman

Collins, in his fascinating autobiography *Anatomy of an Illness*[4], goes even further than this. He believes that humour can actually affect the health of tissue, the rate of healing, and so on. I tend to agree. Certainly, I know that if I am enjoying my work I do it better and, for me, humour is part of that satisfaction. There is no reason for life and work in a nursing home not to be fun.

Money

A built-in drawback from our poorhouse past is our attitude to money. I believe that one of the stereotypes to which old and disabled people are subjected is that of poverty. Very often this is not the case. The accumulation of unspent pension in some forgotten trust account, the eagerness of relatives to help, the philosophy of management and the priorities of local groups, can all become sources of funds for spending on purely pleasurable events and resources. Neither carers nor old people have any responsibility for ensuring that families inherit their relatives' money. We aren't saving for funerals.

Think rich. Ask. Track down sources of funding. They exist. Very often the target of your inquiries will be glad to be asked. Relatives often have trouble designing pleasures for their disabled family member and are glad of your help. Local groups for whom fundraising is the reason for their existence have difficulty sometimes in deciding where they would really enjoy spending money. I consider it an honour and a duty to help them with this problem.

Administration

I believe that one of the nurse's most important roles is as a coordinator of all those activities which impinge upon the life of the old person, especially in the area of extended care. Therefore, we have a responsibility to do much of the staff work that makes the interface between nursing and other professional areas smooth and efficient. For instance, if the old person is going on a bus trip, we need to be sure that he or she is ready on time, suitably dressed and provisioned for whatever might happen.

Nurses have the basic responsibility for patients or residents. This includes proper communication, supervision and planning. We have much to contribute to joint planning exercises where an activity proposal has been canvassed. Will people need a nurse to accompany them on a trip? What pills must go along? Emergency supplies? Insurance? Does anybody need to be notified about what we are planning? Family, doctor, administration? Is there a conflicting appointment?

And this brings other considerations. Which is more important: going to the zoo or to hospital outpatients? My general inclination is to think that bears, lions, picnic sandwiches and no diuretics are very therapeutic.

The beds may be left unmade, the lockers untidy and the record-keeping in shambles, while all these essential things are going on.

Risk-taking

Nurses have a responsibility to ensure the safety and security of the people in their care, and sometimes this gets confused with not taking risks. We sometimes feel we must protect those in our care from any vaguely life-threatening situation, to the extent of protecting them from getting a little bit tipsy at a party, or catching a slight chill at a football match. This notion of safety and security can also come into conflict with the need for self-determination. Yet it need not be so. If the nurse provides this vital element of safety and comfort in the life of the old person, she provides a background from which they can explore and extend their life to its fullest. And this may often require the taking of risks.

Program design should be able to encompass risk to participants. For instance, we have had a broken wrist, a chest infection and a number of falls feature in our vacations away. One woman collapsed from what we thought was heat exhaustion, but the definitive diagnosis turned out to be 'stays that were too tight'.

Quality of dying also becomes an important criterion as we look at the quality of life of older people. Death is probably the area of professional life in which we all have most difficulty. It is certainly the area that our various professional educational backgrounds have dealt with most poorly. It is too large a topic to be dealt with fully here — let it suffice to say that the curing nature of health work should not have the highest priority in our dealings with old people for whom death is an imminent reality. We cannot prevent ageing or death and our care must not suggest that we think otherwise.

Planning properly, caring when we are needed, standing back when we need to stand back, and working as a team with all the players being sensitive, educated and responsible is what it is all about . . .

Summary

Nurses are an essential part of the team that provides an overall health maintenance and rehabilitative service to old people. Their input is essential to any activities program. Their knowledge, sensitivity and the 'generalist' side of their training make them resource treasures. Certainly, the bases for the suggestions in this book are that the term 'activities' be used as broadly as possible; that we all work together — therapists, nurses, domestic staff, families and old people; and that we have a right to enjoy what we are doing and to care for one another while we are about it.

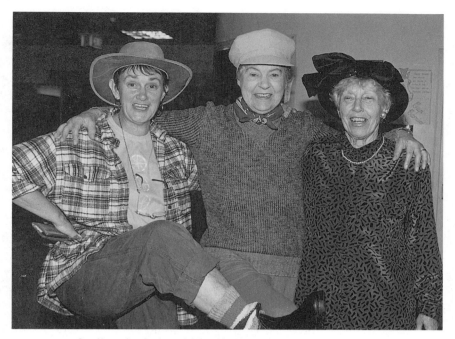

Staff and relatives kick up their heels at a celebration.

References

1. Havinghurst R. *Human Development and Education*. New York: McKay, 1953.
2. Health Department of Victoria: *Regulation of Health Care Agencies and Charities*. 1987; p. 2.
3. Goodman J.Ed. *Laughing Matters*. Saratoga Springs: Sagamore Institute, 1982.
4. Collins N. *Anatomy of an Illness*. Bantam Books Inc, 1979.

Part 2: The Complementary Role of Physiotherapy

by Lyn Grocke*

The idea of promoting independence within a residential setting for frail older people may seem like a contradiction in terms. However, this is exactly the role taken by a therapist. Independence is not an absolute term. Just to be able to relieve pressure in bed or in a chair is, for some people, a precious residual ability.

The team

Care devised from a multi-disciplinary perspective can enrich the lifestyle and experiences of old people in residential care. Intervention that aims to make the most of self-control and relieve the effects of functional loss for residents has been seen to be successful when planned and put into action by health professionals working as a team.

Quality of life for the resident is the paramount aim of all care design. Everyday activities are the focus of intervention for all team members. Through involvement in a range of activity options, the therapist can offer a service which is most relevant to the daily needs of each resident.

The resident

For the residents, the specific knowledge and skills that a therapist applies to problems of mobility may make the difference between being able to choose, without waiting for assistance from others, a space in the sun away from the noise or a seat where the action is. To be included in the pleasantries of the day, the greetings and conversation, presupposes a sitting posture that is comfortable, conveys alertness and allows eye contact. A therapist's expertise can help to get it right.

A visit to a relative or friend's home may provide a welcome break from the communal and routine aspects of a residential care setting. A therapist

---

* Lyn Grocke is the physiotherapist at South Port and is also a member of the team of Carmel Hurst & Associates, a consultancy service for workers in aged care. She provides 20 hours of valuable service to the residents of South Port, although her role as physiotherapist is not always immediately evident. She has been seen involved in many a strange activity, well beyond the realms of the traditional role. Yet her ability to gain the confidence of those requiring her care, and the obvious impact of her services on the level of independence of the residents, suggests there is a hidden agenda in her participation in the life of the home.

can contribute to such a visit by anticipating and preparing for any difficulties in advance. Perhaps the best advice will be the appropriate choice and correct use of a wheelchair for the outing. The important issue is to support relatives and friends in their undertaking as the success and enjoyment of the first visit will significantly increase the chances of it happening again.

The therapist

The role of a therapist in a residential setting is to provide appropriate assessment and care design for the frail older residents. This includes the education of other professionals in various techniques of management and of relatives and friends in order to help them maximise their interactions with the resident.

For a physiotherapist there will always be occasion to provide heat, joint mobilisation, muscle strengthening, gait training and the other tools of a physiotherapist's trade. In a nursing home or hostel where residents enjoy a degree of risk-taking, bruises, strains and sometimes fractures will eventuate and require expert treatment and rehabilitation.

Being part of everyday happenings places a therapist in an ideal position to observe early indicators of deteriorating function. When the energy cost of walking to the dining room has become too much, for instance, it could be because of an infection, an emotional upset or maybe painful feet. Discussion with other team members ensures that appropriate referrals and investigations are made.

Referral protocol is important. The therapist will accept referrals from a wide range of players in the facility including the residents themselves. The therapist will refer in turn to others. The whole concept of multi-disciplinary management is of central importance to a successful outcome.

Conclusion

By complementing the services and activities offered to residents by other staff, families and friends a therapist can influence an individual's ability to maintain a level of independent behaviour by realising their functional potential where possible. For frail older people in residential care the social implications of reaching full potential are great.

PUTTING IT INTO PRACTICE

Chapter 4

Weekly Activities

Olive was a severely disabled woman, whose speech was very laboured and difficult to understand. Her movements were poorly coordinated. Severe muscular contractions confined her to a chair and made sitting for any length of time very difficult. However, she was a very determined person, willing, despite discomfort, to try activities. With aids, she could feed herself and, although messy, she was determined to help herself.

Most activities were thought to be too difficult for her as her upper limb movements were very restricted. Yet one day she was invited to help make some bread. The deftness and strength she applied to kneading the dough were surprising; she loved to cook. With a great sense of determination and love, she made an exotic gateau on the birthday of one of her favourite nurses. She also had a great appreciation of beautiful things. Although outings caused her some discomfort, she loved to go shopping and visit galleries. These activities enabled her to have some pleasure and control over her life, despite her painful disabilities.

I think Olive's story demonstrates the value of involving all those who are interested in activities, regardless of their disabilities.

Weekly activities

The weekly activities form the basic structure of an activity program. They provide predictable, regular events around which participants can plan their week. It is one way in which residents can actively seek to control and influence their daily lives; they can choose whether to take part in activities which interest them, and determine their level of involvement in the selected activities.

Again, it must be remembered that the philosophical and structural frameworks so far described need to be in place to make sure participants' interests and needs are met. The atmosphere of the centre will have a great effect on the level of enjoyment gained from these activities, so it is important that all staff understand and support the involvement of residents in the activity programs. A positive atmosphere is essential and, if everyone feels they contribute to the program and have some sense of ownership for the ideas and events, this is more likely to occur.

Weekly advertising sheets and the daily program board help to keep residents and staff up-to-date. The theme of many activities can be directed by the special events described in Chapter 5, while still retaining the regular program structure.

Guidelines for activities

Group structure

Most of the activities described here take place in small groups. The participants vary. Some groups will probably consist of a strong regular core, while others may form from whoever feels like it on the day. Although a regular core ensures greater friendship and continuity, many participants will have their 'off' days when they will decline to attend. These wishes should be respected. Preferences for companionship should be considered when inviting people to join in group activities, and the selection of participants should reflect each individual's expression of interest in the chosen activity.

Level of participation

Many residents enjoy sitting in a group and watching the fun, giving a hand where they can and offering as much advice as possible. The group atmosphere should encourage socialisation and conversation. For example, while churning ice-cream, the group may like to discuss the ways ice-cream has been made in the past. Others may remember similar activities, comparing it with churning butter, separating cream, or other farm activities. How does manufactured ice-cream compare in taste? Compare favourite flavours and other favourite desserts. Encourage interaction between participants; do not be too directive of the conversation.

If activities are broken down into simple steps, the tasks can then be matched to the abilities of the various participants. In this way, individuals are not barred from taking part by some form of disability. This approach is discussed in Chapter 18.

Flexibility

Flexibility is the key to running these groups. It is important to keep a back-up activity in mind, in case circumstances make the proposed activity inappropriate. Easily prepared table and word games are good back-up activities.

Right to say no

No resident should be forced to join in any of the activities. The right to say 'No' is just as important as the provision of stimulating activities. However, many residents will need plenty of encouragement to join a group and this is best achieved by developing a friendship with each resident, discovering their individual interests and planning a responsive program. Your knowledge of the residents will then enable you to know when to push, and when to let the offer slide.

Sensitivity is needed, yet this is easily lost if the program becomes more important than the people it is there to serve. It is easy to fall into this trap in the excitement and bustle of organising an innovative program. Time must be set aside for chats with individual residents, and the organiser must constantly remind herself of the program's purpose.

Team approach

The activity coordinator may feel she has to be omnipresent and super-human to become friends with all the residents, but the team structure is there to prevent these feelings. We cannot be 'all things to all people'; there will always be residents who irritate us. Yet other staff and volunteers will be able to establish those friendships and encourage participation in the appropriate activities.

New ideas

Always be on the lookout for new activity ideas which can respond to the interests of your residents. Talk to other activity workers and swap ideas. Make contact with cultural associations representing the nationalities of your residents to discover culturally relevant activities and craft ideas. Never limit yourself to the activities listed here, use them instead as a blueprint and a springboard for new ideas which will meet the changing needs of your residents.

Hints for running groups

- Choose a comfortable warm area.
- If concentration is required, find a distraction-free area.
- Be prepared ahead of time, for example, have all the materials ready beforehand.
- Make sure everyone knows each other and you.
- Make the purpose of the group clear to participants.
- Be aware of visual disturbances, such as the effects of glare on cataracts, or reduced visual acuity. Make sure the area has good lighting, use colours with strong contrasts and use large print. Where necessary offer auditory and tactile clues. In games such as bowls, for example, it may help to stand near the target. Peter Rickard's book *Popular Activities and Games for Blind, Visually Impaired and Disabled People* offers some good insights into helping people with visual impairment.[1]

- Be aware of hearing loss. Speak slowly, clearly and at a lower pitch. Use visual cues to demonstrate requirements. Avoid background noise.
- Work alongside group members, rather than leaning over them. Participants, particularly those with some confusion, can then follow your example without feeling they are reduced to the status of students who don't know very much.
- Keep instructions simple and clear.
- Know your participants well so that the right amount of help is given. Get to know each person's tolerance levels for concentration, frustration and tiredness, and be prepared for drop-outs.
- Make sure participants are enjoying their involvement and encourage fun and laughter. A sense of humour is essential. The leader needs to be prepared to make fun of herself.
- Use the activity to stimulate conversation. Discuss variations of the activity, the pleasure it brings, reminisce about similar experiences from the past.
- Collect a library of craft, cookery, and folklore books to use as a source of ideas and recipes.

Activities

The following activities are listed in alphabetical order for easy reference. They have been tested and proved themselves popular, but do be prepared to try new activities as well. If a back-up activity is on hand it doesn't matter if the first activity is not successful. Don't be afraid to fail at times. It is well worth the far greater number of successful new experiences that will result.

- collectors group
- cooking
- crafts and gift-making
- creative art
- creative writing
- discussion groups
- domestic jobs
- drama
- films and videos
- football tipping
- games
- garden club
- hand cream massage
- movement to music
- music appreciation
- outings: drives, community groups
- personal care trolley
- poetry appreciation
- quizzes and word games
- resident of the week
- special community projects
- themes for the week
- woodwork

Collectors group

Value: This activity provides a great social gathering for people with magpie tendencies. Members are also encouraged to make forays into the local community to gather collectible items. The collections can be made into displays, retained by participants or sold for fundraising purposes.

Venue: Activities room or bedroom.

Time allowance: One hour weekly.

Staff ratio: 4–6 residents (very frail) to 1 staff and 1 volunteer.

Stamps

Materials required: inexpensive albums.
Activity ideas:

- sorting and soaking stamps from envelopes
- make individual collections
- decorate covers with stamps — découpage effect
- decorate other items — bins, pot stands, pencil holders — découpage these items
- large wall map — wall hanging
- sorting for charity

Coins

Activity ideas:

- individual collections of coins
- polishing and sorting of coins
- group collection of 5c, 10c, 20c coins
- wood plaques — a tree design can be burnt into the wood with a poker iron, and polished coins stuck on to represent leaves

Other ideas

Other inexpensive items that could be collected:

- postcards — an album for each State
- albums for different countries
- wall map — découpage each State with appropriate cards
- scrapbook — newspaper cuttings about the centre
- keys, badges (metal and cloth), buttons, butterflies, playing cards

Cost: Albums and display card should be the only expense.

Level of participation: This is a popular activity among people who enjoy collecting things. Some fine manipulative skills may need to be intact to perform many of the activities, so some members may prefer to supervise a volunteer to compile their collections.

Cooking

Value: Cooking is familiar, fun, and a good social stimulator. It provides an opportunity for cooks to receive appreciation from eaters, and to enjoy the eating itself.

Cooking facilities: Ideally, a fully equipped kitchenette close to the lounge. Otherwise, frypans and the central kitchen facilities are used. Some basic tools, bowls, spoons, sieve, knives, can be stored in the activity area. Most other equipment can usually be borrowed from the central kitchen, as needed.

Ingredients are obtained from the central kitchen. Special ingredients are purchased with budget funds or resident stall funds.

Venue: Lounge or activities room.

Group size: 2–6 residents.

Time allowance: 1–1½ hours. Actual activity time, 45 minutes.

Staff: Requires one staff member to run the group with volunteer assistance where possible. Prior communication with kitchen staff is essential to plan the use of equipment, oven and hotplates.

Cooking ideas: Favourite recipes, jams and chutneys, meal cookery, followed by lunch together, and special food for celebrations. Cook afternoon tea for everyone.

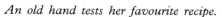

An old hand tests her favourite recipe.

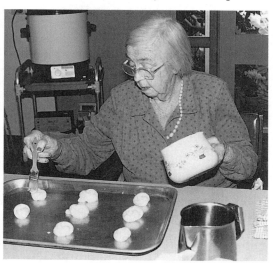

Level of participation: Cooking can be easily adapted to the various abilities of participants. For example, an alert, physically disabled resident may like to be the supervisor, a confused resident could help to chop, mix and sift the ingredients, while an alert, more able resident may want to follow a full recipe individually. Uninvolved observers can be tasters, testers and consumers.

Ideally, there should be a hotplate and oven in the activity area as they enable greater resident participation in the baking process and provide sensory stimulation from cooking aromas.

One-handed hints: Use non-slip matting under bowls and chopping boards. Spiked boards are useful for chopping vegetables and fruit, although it is often simpler to cut the food in half and place the flat surface face down on to the bench. One-handed slicing and chopping can then be quite easy. One-handed sieves, electric beaters, egg separators, potato mashers and teamwork help to overcome most obstacles. (Requests for donations of equipment from relatives, friends and staff are usually successful.)

Cost: Minimal, through using kitchen supplies.

Cooking in a larger institution

As described in Chapter 15, different approaches are required for structuring cooking groups in a larger setting. However, many of the ideas listed here would work very well in smaller settings, too.

Activities room kitchen

Small groups of 3–4 bake cakes, biscuits, slices or scones, prepare morning/afternoon teas or cook and eat a simple lunch. A domestic china dinner service is used for these activities. One staff member needed.

On-ward

A portable oven or frypan is used for group activities for 6–10 residents. Pancakes, hot dogs, homemade soup, pickles and jams, salads, pizzas, biscuits, scones and toasted cheese sandwiches are common fare. Homemade food always brings comments about the difference in taste compared to mass-produced meals.

Entertaining

Entertaining friends is an important part of all our lives, but residential living can make this difficult. The following ideas create opportunities for residents to enjoy sharing a meal or afternoon tea together in a more social atmosphere. Friends from outside should be invited to attend these occasions.

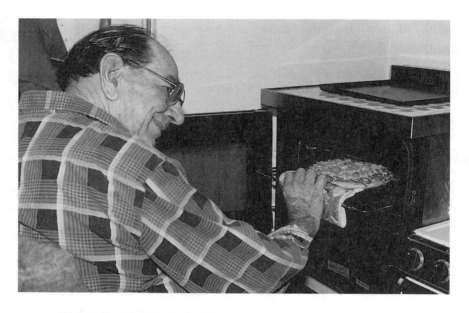

First there is the making then there is the eating!

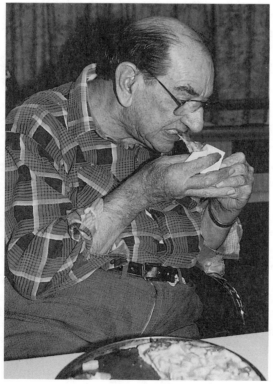

Take-away

Staff go out and buy bulk quantities of take-away food (residents pay for their own), which is eaten in sunrooms or the activities room. Fish and chips are always popular, as are hamburgers, Chinese food, pies and sauce, pizza and take-away chicken.

Barbecues and sausage sizzles

Large and small groups — outdoors whenever weather permits.

Morning and afternoon teas

Venue: Activities room.

Staff ratio: 3–4 residents to 1 staff or volunteer.

Purpose: To entertain 4 residents to a special morning or afternoon tea.

Resources: Fine china tea setting: matching cup, saucer and plate, teapot, sugar basin, jug; cloth; matching paper serviettes; scones.

One such occasion brought together two residents who had worked for years at a local bakery — even though they were on the same floor, neither knew the other was there until they met over this cup of tea. They now meet regularly upstairs for a chat.

There are always such comments as: 'It's a long time since I had a drink out of a lovely china cup' or 'the best thing about that was the lovely cups' — this comment from a man. These teas are usually very relaxed, sharing occasions for residents and are therefore very popular. They can be a worthwhile volunteer project.

Dinner parties and luncheons

Venue: Activities room.

Staff ratio: 12 residents to 3 staff.

Purpose: To entertain 12 residents to a specially prepared three-course meal with all the trimmings: candlelight, music and attractively set tables.

- Usually 6 women and 6 men — staff assist while being part of the party.
- Wine and beer are served with the meal.
- Personal invitations are sent to the residents involved.
- Residents select beforehand from a menu prepared by the main kitchen.
- Dinner parties are held in the evening.
- Luncheons can be held 12–2pm for residents not able to attend an evening function.

Cost: Cost will not be greater than a normal meal.

Crafts and gift-making

Value: In my experience very few residents have been interested in crafts, so craft work is designed to provide residents with the opportunity to give to others: to contribute to fundraising and to make gifts at Christmas time for friends and relatives. Craft work is then a purposeful activity, not a time filler.

Crafts need to be simple, without too many steps, so that quick results are achieved. Unless there are volunteers available to finish work, crafts which require too much machine or detailed finishing should be avoided.

Resources: Any craft books or series of craft magazines can provide good ideas. Volunteers are often experts in certain crafts and will happily teach residents with the help of the activity coordinator. Residents themselves may have skills from their past which can be shared with others.

Consider introducing simple crafts from Asia, India, Europe, South America, Africa and indigenous cultures. Many new craft books describe a great range of effective and simple craft ideas. Invite crafts people to demonstrate their skills so you can learn the crafts and adapt them as necessary.

Venue: Lounge or activities room.

Time allowance: 1 hour.

Group size: Varies with the number interested and available helpers. A one to one ratio is ideal, but 1 helper to 3 residents is workable. Volunteers are essential.

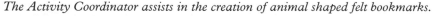

The Activity Coordinator assists in the creation of animal shaped felt bookmarks.

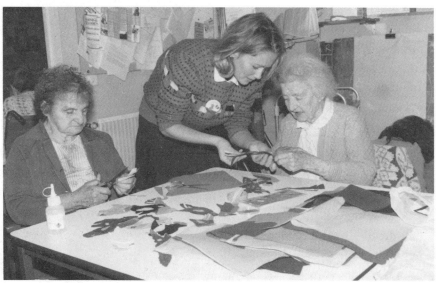

Level of participation: The activities can be shared between residents as their skills allow. Group creativity can be lots of fun and a great shared activity. However, some residents will want to work on their own long-term projects, such as knitting, tapestry, weaving, crochet, or other personal preference. Materials and equipment should be made available for this. There are effective large block tapestries available from most craft shops which are suitable for those with reduced vision and poor manipulative skills.

One-handed hint: Tapestry and some other work can be secured to a wooden frame which is then propped on a stand or clamped to the edge of a table.

Cost: Minimal as materials are usually donated.

It is important to offer residents the opportunity to be involved in giving to family and friends, as so often within the nursing home setting they are care receivers rather than care givers.

The following are some simple ideas for activities which require minimal skill and give quick results.

Pressing flowers

This is very popular, and can be incorporated into the gardening group. Pick the flowers, spread them on absorbent paper, then arrange the sheets between wads of newspaper in a flower press or under heavy books. Press for at least three weeks. The pressed flowers can be used to make cards, pictures or window decorations by ironing them between sheets of waxed paper.

Marbling

Enamel paints are thinned with turps then sprinkled onto the surface of a large shallow tray of water. Cards are dropped onto the surface to absorb the paint. The card can then be glued onto a gift card. Sheets of paper can be used to make wrapping paper.

Pot pourri

Collect scented flowers on walks or outings; invite relatives and friends to bring flowers from their gardens. Spread flowers onto absorbent paper to dry in a ventilated place. Once dry, mix with orris root powder (obtained from craft shops) and spices such as cloves and cinnamon sticks. Cut circles of light fabric, threading a ribbon around the edge to draw fabric into a sachet, and fill with the mixture. Variations: lavender bags, novelty baskets.

Group weaving project

Set up a simple weaving frame. A simple design can be drawn on paper behind the loom as a guide to the weaver, and any interested resident can work at it individually. The loom can be hung at waist level.

Gumnut Christmas wreaths

Collect gumnuts, cut cardboard into circles, glue nuts onto card, then paint the wreath with Estapol and decorate it with Christmas ribbon.

Felt bookmarks

Attractive gifts can be made by cutting felt into animal and bird shapes; each shape can be decorated with smaller pieces of coloured felt to represent wings and markings.

Cooked treats

Truffles, shortbread, gingerbread, homemade chocolates, fudges, jars of preserves with decorated lids.

Other ideas

Residents must be able to work independently with minimum assistance after instruction, as these activities are time-consuming. Volunteer assistance is useful.

- parquetry, leatherwork, simple woodwork
- tapestry — various large-weave canvases
- weaving — on simple frame looms; two shaft weaving; larger scale rug weaving
- foil and copper antiquing
- glass painting
- poker work and wood carving
- glued and padded work — frames, baskets, caneware
- pressed and dried flowers — arrangements, cards, pictures
- jewellery — bead threading, bread dough, leather, nuts
- bread dough novelties, baked and unbaked
- découpage — key holders, pot stands, jars, dishes
- pompom toys
- gathered circles for toys, door stoppers
- glued patchwork — place mats, wall decorations
- caneware novelties decorated with lace, ribbons, flowers
- raffia work

- soap posies and balls, soap-making
- flower-making, using paper or nylon stockings
- candle-making — dipping and marbling
- Christmas decorations

These groups concentrate on making simple personal objects for their own use or to give as gifts to family or friends. Much recycled material is used or residents pay the material costs. If the resident does not wish to keep the article it is sold on a stall to recoup the material costs.

Pottery

Simple handmade pottery using coils, slabs, moulds.

Requirements: Clay, hand tools, storage area, access to a kiln.

Staff: One-to-one assistance is usually required. A volunteer with pottery experience would be most useful.

Ideas: Planters, vases, plates, beads, using simple glazes. Items often have plants bedded in them or contain floral arrangements to complete the project.

Moulded ceramics

This is a worthwhile activity as residents can achieve quality results. Vases, boxes, jugs, ornaments and figurines are common products. It is worth having several moulds of your own, and additional greenware can be purchased from ceramic dealers.

One resident made a jug and bowl set as a wedding present for her niece. She is badly hindered with arthritis, but has found she can cope with this activity and loves doing it.

Equipment and cost: You need to purchase the following basic equipment: clean-up tools, rubber scrubber brushes, various glazes and stains (all available at hobby ceramic dealers). The leader must have some knowledge of the application of glazes.

Creative art

It is worthwhile initially to have a group established by a skilled artist who can be paid to set up the group and provide ideas. An organisation such as Arts Access (see Appendix A) may be able to direct you to an artist. A small group of residents can draw images, colours, flowers and memories. It is important to use good quality crayons and paints and provide gentle relaxing music in the background. Residents require much support and encouragement to use a medium which they have often thought available only to talented artists. Colour, movement, simplicity and self-expression are emphasised.

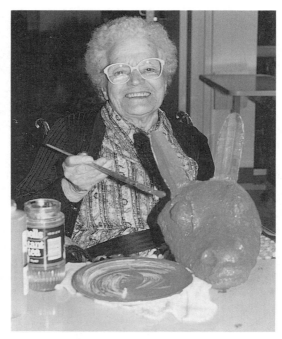

An Arts Access artist works with residents to create masks for the South American Fiesta.

One-handed hints: Non-slip matting or Blu-tack can secure sheets of paper without damaging the corners with tape. Be careful to position paints or crayons within easy reach.

Cost: Initial hire of artist. It may be possible to obtain a grant to fund the artist.

Creative writing

Creative writing can take the form of newsletters, verse and storytelling. You may be fortunate enough to have a resident poet who can write verse for special occasions. He or she may like to work with school children and volunteers in a mutual sharing of skills.

All residents can contribute to a newsletter. It can include gossip, book and television reviews, articles about past and future events, poetry and imaginative prose. A resident could be responsible for editing the newsletter with the help of a volunteer to type the final project. If the home has computer facilities, there are software programs available to arrange newsletter formats and provide graphics, which would contribute greatly to the effectiveness of the final product.

For those who are no longer able to write, volunteer scribes and tape recordings could be used to transcribe stories and events into the written word.

Establish a creative writing group where residents are encouraged to reminisce or tell tales, while the proceedings are tape-recorded. A volunteer could then transcribe the tales into print to enable the residents to become authors.

Cost: paper, photocopying.

Discussion groups

Value: Opportunity for residents to discuss their interests, or history and current events, with other residents in a quiet structured setting. Residents can keep up-to-date with current affairs and it also allows them to talk with others they don't usually mix with. In this way, discussion is both socially and mentally stimulating.

Equipment: Objects or props can be used to help trigger past memories, and to encourage participants to reminisce together. These may include photographs, newspapers, local history books, antiques, and tools which may relate to the past occupations, hobbies and interests of group members.

Venue: Quiet spot.

Group size: 3–6 residents.

Staff: One staff member experienced in group leadership and a volunteer or assistant. Two leaders provide greater resources to encourage residents to participate.

Ideas: Daily newspaper reading and discussion, incorporated with morning tea; discussion of old or recent newspaper stories; reminiscing; situations then and now; personal histories; debates; selected topics of interest. Other ideas are given below.

World trek group

A different country is discussed each month. Stimuli might include inviting a guest speaker, viewing slides and artifacts, listening to music and tasting food allied to the country.

Folk history groups

Usually held weekly, for a few weeks. Discussion centres on photographs and pictures. It may include reading articles and books to stimulate residents' past experience. Music of the time can also be incorporated.

In retrospect

Many local papers have a section describing life 100 years ago, 75 years ago, 50 years ago, 25 years ago. Residents often recall these happenings

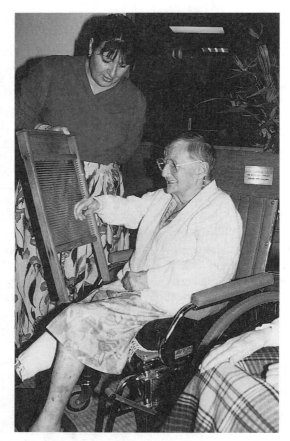

The old wash board triggers many memories.

and actually contribute material to the column. Sometimes a resident gets a mention.

Individual biographies

Some residents may like to record their discussions of their life happenings. Families are often glad to receive a record of their relative's life experiences.

Reading groups

Some residents enjoy listening to short stories and extracts from novels, particularly frail residents who are no longer able to read for themselves. Personal contact is often more acceptable than listening to a tape. Some enjoy a serial reading of a shortened version of a story, perhaps for 15 minutes each day. This provides continuity for the group.

Domestic jobs

A number of residents may like to help with the laundry by sorting socks and stockings and folding small linen, or to assist with plant care and outside sweeping. Often residents enjoy the opportunity to contribute to the general running of the home. They can also help with some food preparations, particularly for special events. These activities can occur at any time as the need arises.

Drama

Value: Opportunity for self-expression.

Drama can be many things — simply play reading, or performances for a concert or theatrical afternoon, skit writing, set production, script writing and performance, or even film-making, if you feel that adventurous! Again, the leader needs to have skills in the area to encourage participants and to develop their talents. A drama expert may need to be invited to help with the group.

Level of participation: It is up to the participants to decide the level of their involvement. Certainly, much fun can be had without professional advice. Some residents may like to attempt script writing, for example, while others may prefer to describe their life experience for someone else to develop into a script. (A professional group of actors developed an excellent play from the experiences of residents at Mt Royal Hospital in Melbourne. It incorporated experiences from past and present to great effect.)

Playback theatre

A Melbourne based group called Playback Theatre has developed a method of performance which is particularly relevant to the aged care setting. Simone Keogh describes her experience of the technique being used in a nursing home.

A Playback Theatre performance is a unique form of improvisational theatre which actively involves the actors and the audience. The people in the audience are invited to tell their stories which are immediately re-enacted by the actors.

While relating their stories, members of the audience are able to regain some feelings of that particular time and also have their story heard without any judgment. A Playback Theatre performance not only provides an accepting mirror for storytellers to see stories enacted; it is also a vehicle for people (in this case, older adults) to share with one another some important times in their lives.

As soon as one storyteller had a story enacted, other residents begin remembering. There is a strong desire to tell and be seen . . . and the feeling of life and vitality is strong.

The performance provides a non-arduous way of reflecting on people's lives and allows participants to celebrate and appreciate what has happened to them as individuals at some particular time or place in their life.

Those who took part in the performance expressed a whole range of emotions and feelings while watching the 'playback'. Many described stories from the depression, and a feeling of camaraderie developed as people shared stories and showed us 'young ones' how it was.

Playback Theatre connects the unique experiences of one person with those of others involved in the event, in a very distinctive style.

Films and videos

Value: A stimulating, entertaining, universally popular activity.

Videos

If you have a video cassette recorder, develop a Movie Buffs' club, whose members can select their favourite movies to watch in the evenings. A staff member on night shift can bring in film videos for a small group of residents who like to stay up late and view the films. I knew of two men who used to sit up till 3am watching movies which the sister on night shift would bring in a couple of times each week. Video hire costs are very small and can be met by participating residents if need be.

Television

Residents who enjoy watching television should be encouraged to keep a television in their own rooms for private viewing. Many residents find the communal area very distracting when watching a favourite show. The communal television should be used with discretion. It can be mesmerising and interfere with other activities. The constant noise of the television can confuse some residents and also disturb hearing-aid users. Residents can agree to watch certain afternoon and evening programs together. The television should never be on unrequested, particularly in the mornings when the programs are geared towards children.

A particular problem is that many residents find the constant interruption of advertisements distracting. If it were not illegal, it would be worth recording good programs and replaying them with the advertisements edited out. We had one very alert resident who lived through the times of the Australian *Waterfront* series. It was set where he used to work and live, yet he did not watch the series as he found that the constant interruption of advertisements made following the storyline impossible.

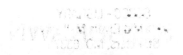

In-house video

Some larger centres have an in-house television channel which allows a selection of videos to be channelled through to the centre's televisions.

Films

Videos do not replace 16mm films, however. Many residents cannot focus their full attention on a movie presented on the small screen, and daytime viewing of television movies is difficult because of the many distractions.

It is most worthwhile to hire good 16mm films to show to a large group as a daytime activity. Popular musicals of the 1930s and 1940s are always well received. The large screen and special effort involved in arranging the audience help to make the viewing of the film a special event. A short interval with popcorn and chips can add to the atmosphere.

Resources: Free films can be obtained from the State Film Library, although their quality and interest level is sometimes limited.

Film distributors are easily found in the telephone directory and supply many of the old MGM 'greats' and up-to-date films. I have found the Movielink Film Distributions particularly good. They supply excellent quality prints of many wonderful old musicals and films. Hire costs start at $50 for the old MGMs, increasing for the newer films. They also deliver at a reasonable cost (see Appendix C).

Equipment: A standard 16mm projector and large screen is sufficient for the older movies. The newer movies require the extra hire of a cinemascope lens and a wide screen or sheets. Although this requires extra effort, it is a special treat to view films on such a large scale. Most local libraries or schools will lend their equipment, or projectors can be hired from many film and projector distributors.

Venue: Any room which can be darkened adequately. If the entire room cannot be darkened, darkening the screen end will still enable good viewing.

Time allowance: Most films are about 100 minutes long. 10am to 12 noon is the best time to view, when residents are most alert.

Staff: One staff member is needed to organise the activity, while nursing staff are required to help get everyone up in time, and to arrange the audience.

Outings to see films at a cinema are an alternative, though this means limiting the group size. Few cinemas provide easy wheelchair access to the theatre or toilets. Some which are accessible to wheelchairs offer a special pensioner rate film and luncheon which can make a very pleasant outing.

Football tipping

For football, soccer, rugby, etc. Competition runs throughout the sporting season. Residents each have a fixture card on which they mark the teams they think will win each week. A tally of weekly scores is kept, with a major prize for the one who picks the most winners over the season. Cards are usually marked at lunchtime on Friday. This creates rather a buzz in a usually quiet setting as residents argue over who is going to win. It provides quite an interest for some who are not involved in any other activity.

Games

Value: Socialisation, recreation and physical exercise.

Equipment: Board games, for example, scrabble, draughts, Yahtsee, cards, dominoes, Concentration, backgammon, Trivial Pursuit. Quoits, carpet or plastic sheets with scoring circles, beanbags, coins, balls, skittles, carpet bowls, walking sticks, darts, hookey board.

Venue: Lounge or activities room.

Group size: Varies from 2–4 to large groups in teams.

Time allowance: $^{1}/_{2}$–1 hour. The game could be a spontaneous request for a quick activity among a few people. Alternatively, some preparation will be required for team sports. Here, the teams could play one game or move around a selection of three or four activities, to provide more interest and entertainment. With a little more preparation the games could be turned into a special social event, by setting up a casino-style environment and playing a range of gambling games; perhaps for a games evening (club night). Use prizes, of course, rather than money. (A police raid may be a new experience, but not really to be desired!)

Staff: For active games, it is best to have 2 organisers, either volunteer or staff.

Level of participation: Participation will vary with the game, ranging from simple throwing games for the less active to competitive team sports for those brave enough to join in.

Note: The involvement of school children in these activities encourages residents to participate more freely on the children's behalf.

Bowls

Men's and ladies' indoor bowls

Weekly groups. Team competitions, some mixed group sessions, a singles championship and bi-monthly competitions against another local centre.

Greens bowls

Able and interested residents participate in weekly competitions on a local green. Players also visit other local bowling clubs for social days.

Dice games

Apart from the usual board and table games, here are a few others.

Crown and anchor

Players: 2 or more.

Equipment: A large board or card divided into 6 sections and numbered from 1 to 6; 3 dice, a shaker and a supply of counters.

Rules:

1. To start, each player throws the dice — highest scorer becomes banker.
2. Bets are made by placing counters on a particular number on the board.
3. When all bets are placed the banker throws the 3 dice and pays according to the following:

Score	Pay out
single	stake back plus one stake
doubles	stake back plus twice stake
trebles	stake back plus three times stake

Bets on any number not shown on the dice are collected by the banker. After 10 throws the banker should change.

High dice

Players: 2 or more.

Equipment: 2 dice.

Rules:

1. Each player tries to beat the first shooter.
2. The first shooter has several advantages over other players: (a) he/she wins all the ties (b) the first shooter automatically wins if he/she throws 2 sixes.
3. Decide the first shooter by a throw of the dice — the highest scorer starts.
4. Change the first shooter after 5 rounds or less if need be.

Rotation

Players: 2 or more.

Equipment: 2 dice, pencil and paper to score.

Rules:

1. Each player takes turns trying to get a certain number on each throw of the dice.
2. Each has 11 chances (or rounds) to score. First round each player tries for a 2, second round for a 3, etc. The sum of the dice equals the number.

3. If you succeed you receive the score equalling the number tried for; if not, there is no score.

Pig

Players: 2 or more.

Object: The first to score 100 or more points.

Equipment: One die, paper and pencil to score.

Rules:

1. Each player throws the die — the highest scorer starts.
2. Each player may throw the die any number of times as long as he/she doesn't throw a 1.
3. If a 1 is thrown, the player's turn is over and he/she loses that round of points.
4. If the player decides to end the turn before throwing a 1, he/she scores all the points from that round of throws.

Table games

Most table games are suitable though some may need their rules simplified to shorten the length of play. Others may need some adaptation to accommodate visual and motor impairments. The Royal Institute for the Blind and the Association for the Blind both offer good advice and also act as distributors for some of the commercially available adapted games.

Commercially available games include:

- Large scrabble, produced by Selchow and Richter Company; Bay Shore, New York, 1982.
- Raised dominoes and backgammon, produced by the Royal National Institute for the Blind; Great Portland, London.
- Large playing cards.

A useful text for adapting games and activities is Peter Rickard's *Popular Activities and Games for Blind, Visually Impaired and Disabled People.*[1]

Active games

Value: These games encourage physical exercise, both from the activity itself and the resultant laughter. Competitors should not take the games too seriously, but see them as another chance to let their hair down and have fun. They should definitely only be played by those who actively choose to be involved.

Staff: A staff member and volunteer are needed, and any passersby can act as cheerleaders and coaches and add to the crazy atmosphere.

Level of participation: These games appeal to some more than others.

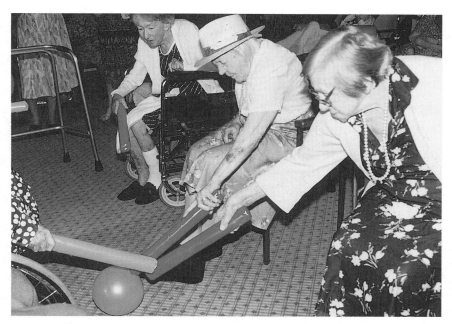

A game of hockey in full swing. Note soft battens and ball reduce risk of injury.

Physical disabilities should not prevent people from taking part, but personal preferences may. Again, the involvement of children can encourage people to participate.

Hockey

Two rows of teams face each other seated in chairs with arms; each player has a walking stick turned upside down. Use a large lightweight ball, and walking frames as goals at each end. Each team member attempts to hit the ball towards one end while preventing the opposite team from moving the ball to the opposite end. Place strategic players at the ends of rows as goal attacks and goal keepers. (Remember to consider ease of swing of one-handed people when setting up teams.)

Rules: Keep sticks low and out of contact with opponents' legs; keep bottoms on seats.

Staff: Requires a staff member or volunteer for each team as coach and cheerleader.

Soccer or football

Play as for hockey, kicking a light soccer ball with feet.

Goal-kicking and handball

Use a laundry skip frame as a handball target, and a plastic football. Using Blu-tack, attach white strips of card as goalposts onto a wall; kick a soft football at the posts to score goals and points.

These are ideal activities at Grand Final time.

Pitch and toss

Mark a carpet piece with concentric circles to form a target. The centre is worth 50 points, the next circles 20, 10 and 5 points. Seat players around the target in a circle; throw washers, coins or small beanbags to score.

Cricket

Use a plastic sheet with a grid drawn on it — 9 squares with different results in each: 1 run, 2 runs, 3 runs, a six, a four, run out, lbw, clean bowled, caught, etc. Two teams; each player has three throws of the beanbag to score for his or her team.

This approach can be adapted to other sports such as baseball, football and tennis, by changing the form of scoring which is displayed on the sheet.

Volleyball

Use a balloon as a volleyball. Set up a rope between two chairs to form a net. Teams face each other and hit the balloon to keep it off the ground and over the net. A score is made if the ball falls to the ground on the opposite side.

Relays

Two teams sit in rows facing each other and pass objects along the row, aiming to beat the other team. Use beanbags, balls or fine manipulation objects, for example, use tweezers to remove object from jar before passing it on; tie bows; put on hats, aprons, jewellery; shake hands.

Crossball

Two teams, each with two rows of team members facing each other. Throw beanbags or balls across to team members sitting opposite, aiming to beat the other team.

Tunnelball

Two rows, seated in chairs one in front of the other; knock ball between legs with walking stick or hands.

Round robin

Set up three games — board, quiz or sport — and rotate teams at the end of each game. Total the scores at the end for each team. Requires 3–4 leaders.

Carpet bowls

Members can play as individuals or as teams, following the general rules of lawn bowls. Ensure participants can reach the floor from their chair, and that they are well supported as they lean forward (footplates up).

Note: Think of a sport, then think of a way of modifying it for wheelchairs and frail bodies.

Garden club

Value: Gardening is a very familiar activity; most people enjoy plants and have some expertise in the area. It is also relatively easy to grade the activity to suit varying abilities. The plants themselves have a significant effect on the environment — indoor plants and attractive garden areas give much visual pleasure as well as a resource for activity.

Equipment: Long-handled garden tools (or tools which can be adapted by the woodwork group) and hand tools. Some tools may need to be purchased, some can be borrowed from the maintenance department. Often relatives and volunteers will have a few tools they are willing to donate or lend.

Resources: Contact your Horticultural Society or garden society. They may be able to send a volunteer to run a number of sessions and give talks; they may also provide tools and seeds. This is an excellent way to establish an ongoing garden club. Invite interested staff, volunteers, school groups and relatives to join residents in forming a club which meets regularly. Such a club can then become a member of the Horticultural Society, gaining access to continuing advice, ideas and resources.

Venue: Choose between the activities room, garden or lounge, depending on the size of the group and the activity, and the extent of mess caused by the activity.

Time allowance: 1–2 hours.

Staff: Any staff member or volunteer who is a keen gardener can run this group. One staff member is required to oversee the group to ensure participation, safe positioning of residents, supply of equipment and co-ordination of events. However, volunteers provide a strong source of input and direction for this group. They will often bring cuttings, pass on hints and skills, and lend equipment. Join forces with the local schools to enable residents to work alongside the students and share skills.

It is important to establish good communication with the gardening department of the home, in order to coordinate activities and planting sites and organise the supply of tools and seedlings.

Projects

Design garden plots; establish a vegetable or herb garden; design raised garden beds. Plants could be grown and sold to staff and relatives to create a small industry.

- propagation of seeds, bulbs, cuttings, seedlings
- planting raised beds and window boxes
- miniature succulent gardens
- hanging baskets
- herbs — growing and drying — mint, parsley, rosemary, pot pourri herbs
- making pot pourri novelties
- making Australian pot pourri from gumnuts, leaves, eucalyptus
- moulding and painting garden frogs and gnomes
- covering pots with shells or tiles
- pottery — making pots and vases
- floral arrangements, dried and fresh

Two keen gardeners tend the indoor and outdoor plants.

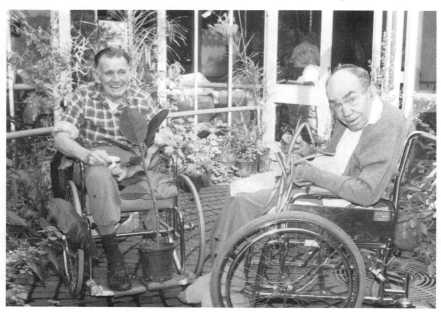

- pressing and drying flowers — use for cards, pictures, wall plaques
- collecting gumnuts, seeds and bark — for wall hangings and novelties
- terrariums/bottle plants
- making salads with home-grown vegetables
- jam and pickle-making in season
- making mint sauce
- visiting speakers and demonstrations
- videos on aspects of gardening
- visiting local gardens of interest
- walking in the Centre's gardens; picking and arranging flowers
- bird feeders to hang in trees outside windows.

A useful reference for gardening is *Esther Dean's Gardening Book: Growing without Digging*[2], which describes a method of gardening using straw and newspaper. It has particularly useful information on raised garden beds, those, for example, which are built on framed table tops or in a garden bed framed with sleepers or bricks to raise the level of the working surface.

Level of participation: Some residents prefer to offer advice and direction rather than do hands-on work, particularly with bigger jobs. However, many residents enjoy striking cuttings, planting seeds and seedlings, and potting plants, whether they can only assist a volunteer or do the full task themselves.

Hand cream massage

All residents have individually marked pots of hand cream which are circulated to all available staff and volunteers, who then spend time each week chatting with residents and massaging their hands, and feet, if so desired. No resident is forced to join in but most, including the men, enjoy the contact and the time to chat more intimately, as well as the opportunity to improve their skin. Relatives particularly are encouraged to participate in this activity, which provides a safe, acceptable opportunity for touching.

Value: Many residents have very little physical contact with others, particularly with their families and friends. This is a relaxed safe way of providing such contact.

Movement to music (see also Chapter 8)

Value: Exercise to maintain physical function, music to provide pleasure and fun.

Equipment: Cassette player; tapes with a variety of music for different exercises; scarves; balloons; percussion instruments; streamers; large piece of lightweight fabric.

Venue: Lounge or activities room.

Group size: Small or large groups.

Time allowance: 30–45 minutes.

Staff: At least 1 staff member with appropriate training and any other volunteers available. Volunteers can help to add an atmosphere of fun.

Exercises for head, neck, shoulder, arm, trunk, hip, knee and ankle are achieved by using the theme of the music: football songs and marching music for lower limbs; gentle relaxing music for head, neck and shoulders; piano music for finger exercises; ballet music for large smooth trunk movements. Use floating music and balloons or scarves to exercise upper limbs and trunk. Hitting balloons is surprisingly popular. Scarves should be lightweight so they float to the music. A large piece of lightweight material can also be used — group members sit in a circle and hold onto the edge of the material. They can then make waves or roll balloons around to the music.

Music appreciation (see also Chapter 8)

Value: To provide opportunity for residents to enjoy and explore their individual tastes in music. Discussion and special requests are encouraged.

Equipment: Reasonable stereo system. You will need a portable cassette and compact disc player which produces good sound and allows for versatility of venue. Access to a music library is necessary. Staff and volunteers may like to bring compact discs and tapes for specific themes.

Venue: Somewhere quiet and restful, removed from the general area.

Group size: Small but variable; those interested in the specific style of music.

Staff: This group is easily run by 1 person, preferably a volunteer.

Ideas: Classical, jazz, country, and special interest groups.

Music-oriented groups in the larger institution

The following additional suggestions are suitable for larger institutions, particularly those in country regions.

Community singing

This can involve a group of up to 40 residents in a weekly event. The program can include a guest artist for seasonal events and a segment of residents' choices. Residents can meet weekly for singing as well as some percussion activity. Two staff needed. (*The Ulverscroft Large Print Song Book*[3] is produced in both word and music editions.)

Organ recital

A portable electronic organ and a musical volunteer can circulate throughout the centre to give recitals. This is very popular, especially with very frail residents.

Visiting performers

A wide variety of artists, choirs and bands can be invited to visit the centre throughout the year.

Visits to musicals and concerts

Parties may attend performances of popular musicals, orchestral concerts, organ recitals, and visiting artists. These productions are always enjoyed and provide a talking point for days afterwards. Residents are often invited to dress rehearsals, usually free. It is much easier to take dependent people, especially those in wheelchairs, when the theatre is less crowded.

Outings

These are included here simply as a suggested weekly activity. Outings are discussed in greater detail in Chapter 6.

Drives

Small groups of residents may enjoy going for a drive each week. The destination can be varied, afternoon tea can be taken to consume on the bus, or ice-creams bought along the way.

Equipment: Wheelchair bus, borrowed from the council or local hospital.

Venue: Parks, beach front, suburbs with special interest, nearby countryside, city and surrounds — depending on the locality of the home.

Group size: Depends on the capacity of the bus and the number interested.

Time allowance: 1–1½ hours. No longer, to avoid toilet stops. Longer trips where participants disembark are described in Chapter 6.

Staff: Staff member to supervise trip. Volunteer driver. Extra staff to load and unload residents at the centre.

Participants: The group can be varied, from the very alert to quite low-functioning residents.

Community activities

One or more residents may want to attend activities in the local community. The local government municipal recreation officer will be able to direct you to groups which exist in the community. These may include neighbourhood house groups, recreational activities or specific classes. Car transport may be all that is needed for such small groups. This may lead to a number of different residents regularly going out at different times during the week. Volunteer drivers can assist greatly with these activities. The importance of community involvement in these groups cannot be overemphasised. (See Chapter 9 for community resource information.)

Personal care trolley

Decorate a trolley with an attractive cloth and stock it with skin care, make-up and manicure items. Use good quality products which are non-allergic and have no perfumed additives. Staff can be trained by a product representative from the store of purchase when beginning the program. Ask about suitable regimes for older women. The trolley can be made available to any resident for special occasions with one-to-one attention, or a volunteer on a weekly basis could give some residents a real morale booster. It can be made available to very frail people for gentle hand massage as stimulation.

Directions for use

1. Before doing anything, wash hands.
2. Check that you know which creams to use and in which order.
3. For hygienic reasons, never use your fingers to dip into make-up containers — use plastic spoons, cotton wool and cotton-tipped applicators.
4. Finally, be sparing. Make-up is highly concentrated and very expensive. People do not want to be 'over-painted'.
5. Remember, while you work, talk with the resident; the session should be fun for both of you.

Basic requirements

- gentle cleansing cream
- clarifying lotion
- moisturiser
- soft foundation
- face powder
- lipstick
- perfume
- greaseless body lotion or hand cream

- mirror
- small bowl and soft towels
- container for used cotton wool, spoons, etc
- plastic spoons
- cotton wool balls
- cotton-tipped applicators
- manicure equipment
- bowl of rose water with marbles to roll about while hands are soaking

Poetry appreciation

This may be a small group of residents who would enjoy reading and writing poetry and ballads together. A volunteer could be responsible for the collection of material.

Quizzes and word games

Value: Intellectual stimulation, socialisation and fun.

Equipment: Blackboard, chalk and stand. Quiz and word game books.

Venue: Lounge or activities room.

Group size: Any number. A casual set-up, where everyone can see the board and hear from where they sit, encourages participation from those who dislike being relocated to join activities.

Time allowance: 30–45 minutes.

Staff: One staff member, or volunteer, is required to run a quiz. Quizzes are more fun if other staff and volunteers participate whenever possible, even if only in passing.

Level of participation: Quizzes can be varied to suit the interests and abilities of residents.

Ideas: Most word game and quiz books found in good bookstores have a wealth of ideas, for example, crosswords, general knowledge, guessing games.

Last-minute ideas

1. Find smaller words from a larger one.
2. Hangman (see page 143 if you're unfamiliar with this game).
3. Continuous words: choose a category, for example, animals; use last letter of previous word to think of the next word, for example, kangaroo — orang-outang — gnu.
4. Fives: divide a board into 6 by 6 sections; choose 5 categories across

and 5 alphabet letters down. The group must think of five items in each section. See example following.

	ANIMAL	CITY	FLOWER	FOOD	CAREER
B	bat beaver bison	Bendigo Bathurst		bread	
C	cat		Photo 16	cheese	catering
T			tulip		teaching
N		Newcastle			
L	lion leopard				

5. Alphabet categories: the group chooses a category such as sport, then goes through the alphabet calling out as many sports as they can that start with A, then B, C and so on, throughout the alphabet. To create a bit more fun, a leader could select answers before the game and make the group guess her word, before moving on to the next letter. This encourages greater participation (and cheating by the leader is allowed).

The following ideas need more preparation.

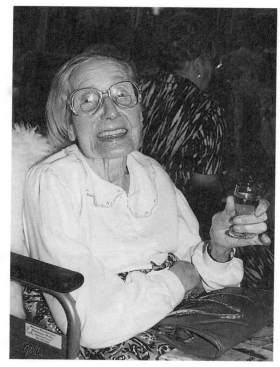

A happy hour could occur daily rather than weekly!

Crosswords

It is best to have a grid set up permanently, onto which a crossword can be drawn. Make sure the answers are on hand so the leader can offer extra clues if the group is struggling to find the answer.

Trivial Pursuit

For a large group, clip the board onto the blackboard, use Blu-tack to move the tokens, divide into two teams and give a wedge for each correct answer.

Pairs

1. Match leading ladies with leading actors in films.
2. Word associations, using a quiz book for ideas.

Who am I?

Use *Who's Who*, encyclopaedias and magazines as resource material. A volunteer could be invited to devise character descriptions. Each description is read out slowly so teams can guess the person's name before it is completed.

Photograph recognition quiz

Use magazines as a resource for pictures of people, flowers, cities, monuments. Individuals or teams can guess the identity of each photograph.

Baby photo quiz

Collect baby photos of staff, residents and volunteers to create a competition. Run the quiz for two weeks, allowing anyone interested to enter. Give prizes to the winners.

Modified charades

Participants are given a card with the name of a profession, animal, food or object to act out to the rest of the group. The group has to guess the answer.

Musical quiz

Play pieces, asking participants to guess the musician, singer or writer, the next line in the song, or the film it is from. Use cassettes, records or, if able, play the piano.

Musical themes

Select a theme, asking participants to think of songs which match the theme. For example, songs which include first names, or a colour, bird, season or time of year.

A list of song titles which can be used for these quizzes can be found in Appendix F. Further quiz ideas are included in Chapter 8.

Local area quiz

Invite a resident, relative or volunteer who has good knowledge of the area to compose a quiz about the area's history, people, events and landmarks.

Other creative ideas for quizzes can be found in commercially available quiz and word game books.

TV show games

Value: Although the games described here take some preparation time, they are well worth it for the fun and stimulation they create. A volunteer may be able to do the research and much of the preparation.

Family feud/blankety blanks

Before the game, survey residents, staff and volunteers for the first answers which come to mind to selected questions. Set up a panel of 2 teams, 3 in each. The teams must try to guess the most popular answers to the same questions, scoring highest if they match the most popular answers. This is a particularly good game as it does not require intellectual brilliance to succeed.

It's academic/sale of the century (Or other quiz show format)

Direct the quiz questions to a panel; if the panel can't answer the question, open it up to the audience.

The price is right (Or other shopping game)

Obtain a selection of everyday items to price. Variations can include the nearest correct guess, ordering items from cheapest to dearest, and grouping items of similar price. Good orientation game.

Wheel of fortune

Use the commercially available game, adapting it to a lager group.

Adapt new games

It is worth suffering through a few game shows on television to gain more ideas.

Resident of the Week

Each week one person may be chosen by staff as resident of the week. This may mean that the selected resident wears an identifying badge. Everyone is then encouraged to affirm that person's worth throughout the week, letting them know why they have been chosen. Their qualities are emphasised and some special services may be offered to that individual during the week. This may mean granting a specific wish to the resident. Throughout the year each person living in the centre should be elected at least once.

Value: The 'Resident of the Week' program ensures that every person receives some special attention and affirmation beyond the usual care offered by staff. As all residents are selected at some time, it helps to foster a sense of well-being; everyone gets a chance to feel special. Each person is affirmed simply for being the person they are. There is definitely no manipulative intention to change behaviour.

Special community projects

Many one-off projects are very worthwhile. They suit particularly those residents who prefer to do a task-oriented project to help someone else.

They are also useful for encouraging residents to contribute to the lives of others.

Recipe book

As a fundraising venture, recipes can be collected from residents, relatives, friends and staff and collated into book form. Residents can be involved in the collection, the writing, artwork, photocopying and collating, marketing and selling of the final product.

General collating work

Some residents may like to volunteer to help with the centre's clerical work. Some enjoy collating, hole punching and stapling now and then. You may find those who usually decline involvement in most leisure activities may actually prefer such specifically work-oriented, purposeful activity. It must definitely be a totally voluntary activity, where the need is made known and people are given the opportunity to offer their services freely.

Child sponsorship

A number of residents may like to pool resources to sponsor a child through an overseas aid organisation. Participants may want to donate funds directly, or commit themselves to fundraising projects on behalf of the child.

Themes for the week

Value: A theme can be selected to direct the week's activities, enhancing a sense of purpose and direction in the program. These themes provide a good base for reality orientation which will affect the entire population of the centre, and they avoid the classroom approach which is not always appropriate to a home environment. Food, clothing, displays, guest speakers, demonstrators, performers, crafts, outings, can all be centred around a special theme. The themes can be selected by the residents.

Such 'theme' weeks will allow you to discover the interests and skills of residents and volunteers, particularly if followed by informal discussion with residents about the activities they liked best. A card file of residents' abilities and interests can be kept for future reference.

The following are some suitable themes.

Reminiscing

Discussions comparing past and present; Do you remember when . . . ?; collecting 'old wives' tales'; creating a display of old photographs; old-style cooking; clothing; crafts; spinning yarns; old-time dancing; performances; a visit to a museum, historic building, or reconstruction of the past such as an old gold mining town or folk town; a tour of the participants' home ground. A good resource to trigger discussions is *Family Memories* by Bob Price.[4]

Animals

Discuss favourite animals, old pets, working animals. Discuss the care of the resident cat, dog and budgies. Invite relatives to bring in their pets. Organise an animal show with competitions. Go to the zoo or invite the Zoo Education Service to visit — they will bring animals for the residents to handle (make sure they bring a snake), and show slides of the zoo. Visit a wildlife sanctuary. Invite an expert in the care of certain animals to visit, for example, from the Budgerigar Council, Police Dog Squad, an animal farm, Police Horse Academy (make sure they bring the horses inside), Guide Dog Association or Hearing Dog Service.

Gardening

Show slides, visit famous gardens, discuss own gardens, favourite flowers, plants, planting hints. Organise flower displays and flower arrangement demonstrations and lessons. Invite gardening experts to speak. A regular

This visiting chook finds a friend.

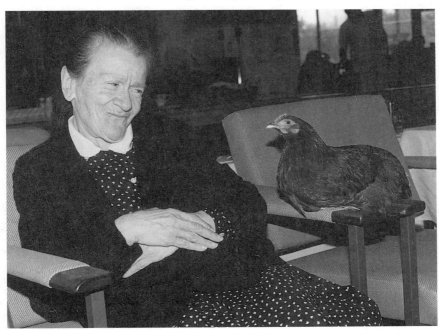

gardening club could be established following a week of special emphasis on gardening.

The arts

Invite exhibitions to visit the home. Go to galleries, the theatre, craft displays, drama workshops, theatrical and musical performances by professionals, amateurs or school groups. Invite experts in painting, sculpture, pottery, copperwork and other specialised crafts to visit and demonstrate their skills. Visit workshops, for example, a major tapestry workshop, then visit any public building which may display one of their works.

A theme week such as this may be a good opportunity to invite an artist to assume the role of Artist-in-Residence (see Chapter 9).

Countries of the world

Plan in-house vacations to other countries. Cook and eat food from the different cultures, display their dress and art, invite speakers and dancers, show films and celebrate their special events (see Chapter 5).

Current events

Follow current events such as the America's Cup, football and cricket seasons, political elections, International Year themes, centenary events, current plays, musicals and films. These can all be used to direct activities and events. Be alert and respond to the events which surround you.

Seasons

At the beginning of each season a special focus can be made on the time of year. Activities may include: creating displays of spring or summer flowers, or autumn leaves; gardening which relates to the seasons; outings to gardens to observe the changing effects of different seasons; reminiscing about events that occurred in specific seasons of the year; old and new ways of dealing with the extremes of weather conditions.

Woodwork

Value: Familiar activity with very tangible outcome.

Tools   are limited to basic hand tools, some donated by residents and volunteers, while others are purchased from budget funds. Access to maintenance department tools is also useful.

Materials: Wood is purchased with budgetary funds; some donations may be received.

Venue: Sheltered area outside and/or activities room.

Group size: 2–6.

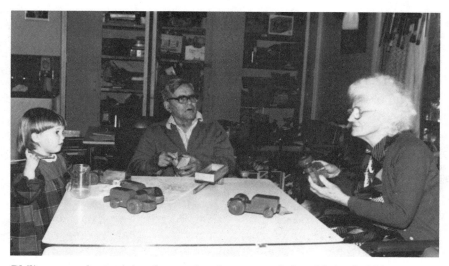

Philippa, aged two, joins the woodwork group to help add the finishing touches to some wooden toys. (Philippa painted with water.)

Time allowance: One hour.

One-handed hints: Clamps of all sizes are useful to secure work. Simple jigs can be made with blocks of wood, clamps, dowel posts and nails to enable sawing, drilling, sanding and painting with only one hand. For example, a block of wood with a number of dowels inserted along it can act as a support while sanding and painting wheels or flat objects.

Staff: One staff member, and a volunteer with woodwork experience. Maintenance staff are sometimes asked for tools and advice.

Project ideas: Outdoor furniture, garden boxes, repair of children's toys and furniture for the local creche or kindergarten, simple children's toys. There may be a local person who makes toys and would like residents to sand and varnish the work.

Level of participation: To simplify the task, order wood cut to measure for the project. Sanding and painting provide the most activity. Volunteers and any abler residents work together to construct the project. A sense of working together and pooling skills is then encouraged.

The very frail older person

Time and again, activity workers tell me that their residents are just so much frailer than those of other nursing homes. 'Things have changed over the last few years,' they say, 'the residents in your book are more alert and active than ours. We can't do those things here.' Yes, people in nursing homes are frailer — in all nursing homes throughout Australia —

but that has not prevented many more nursing homes from introducing creative, lively activities into their centres. As a consultant working with activity workers in nursing homes, I often hear these comments. Even so, a few months later, the same activity workers find they can introduce just about all the activities suggested in this book. Certainly, the changed funding criteria does mean that nursing homes do now house many frail people. But it does not mean that the very frail older person cannot enjoy the odd party, musical event or simple activity for short periods of time.

By way of definition, the very frail person is likely to have very little communication, able to only cry out or mumble incoherently. She may have no functional movement and may only tolerate staying out of bed for short periods.

When working with very frail older people it is essential to have a good social history (see Chapter 17), as this enables you to look past the frailty and to consider the depth of human experience that the frail older person holds within them. This is important for a number of other reasons. A very dependent person is just that — dependent on staff to ensure a sense of quality of life. The resident may not be able to communicate her wishes and will rely on your knowledge to ensure that she is involved in appropriate activities. With knowledge you can select activities which you know she will love rather than ones which will inflict frustration and irritation. You will know when to select passive activities which offer soothing, gentle reassurance.

It is also important to respect a person's right to refuse group activities. The social history will help you to know if a person has sought out company or has preferred to remain alone or with just one or two friends. Recognise too, the low energy levels and pain that a very frail person may be experiencing. This will often mean that there are times when peace and rest is the best activity. Perhaps the reassurance of a curled up cat on the bedcover may be enough comfort between nursing care activities. Here again, the frail person is very reliant on especially gentle and high quality care for all their personal care activities. The nurse will play a very important role in the quality of life of a very frail person.

For example, in one nursing home I worked with recently, the Director of Nursing gave especial encouragement to a nurse to spend as much time as possible offering massage, reading the Bible and praying with a woman who was known to have a Christian faith. That woman died having received a great deal of quiet love and reassurance. Nothing more important could have been offered.

Activity suggestions

Below is a list of activities which are usually appropriate for a very frail person. However, be guided in your selection by your knowledge of that person's social history.

General activities

Those who are very frail and dependent in most areas of personal care, and have some substantial communication difficulties, can often still contribute significantly to cooking, singing, music and other simple activity groups — whether it be as an observer, or to do simple mixing and chopping or to test the food that has been cooked.

It is important to focus activities across the spectrum of sensory abilities: sight, sound, touch, scent, taste and movement.

Music

The benefits of music should never be underestimated. Even the frailest residents can benefit from all aspects of music, including movement to music, quiet listening, singing and musical percussion. Consider employing a music therapist for a few hours of your program. A music therapist can introduce a wonderful range of musical activities which can cater especially for frail older people.

Despite her frailty, music transforms this woman.

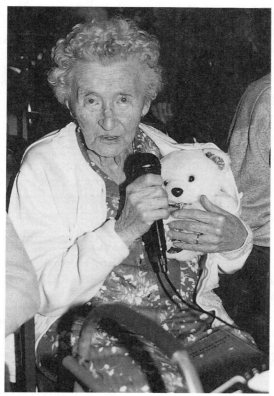

Massage

Many Directors of Nursing are introducing training in massage techniques for their staff as they find it has great benefit for very frail people. Head, shoulder, hand and foot massage can quickly sooth the distressed resident. A fuller massage can occur as part of personal care to increase circulation and preserve skin integrity. For others, it is simply a chance to enjoy spending time with another person and experience gentle touch. This is important as many older people do not find many opportunities to touch and be touched in a secure environment.

Facial and manicure care

A personal care trolley creates a very special occasion out of a simple task of personal care. If a tea tray is converted by covering it with floral material, it can then be decorated with a bowl of pot pourri, perfume, and attractive china dishes. A small dish of marbles, with scented water, can be used to prepare each hand for manicure. Stores of low allergy facial products, manicure equipment and disposable appliques can be stored on the bottom shelf, hidden by the skirt of the trolley.

Cooking

Cooking should be encouraged, as it provides a valuable opportunity for a multitude of sensory stimulation. Ideas include afternoon tea items, soups, jams and chutneys, simple chocolate making and other confection-ery. The frail person may sit and observe the activity or simply taste the results. Some, given a vegetable knife and fruit or vegetables, will cut automatically.

Celebrations

The person may enjoy the music, food and atmosphere of a celebratory day for short periods. It is surprising how well some people can manage finger food at a party even though they would otherwise be limited to a very soft diet (see Chapter 5).

This is Your Life Book

Invite a relative or volunteer to collect any photographs and newspaper cuttings etc to compile into an album about the person's life. Staff and relatives can then use it as a tool to help the person reflect upon and value their past life and to have it acknowledged by staff.

Camera and photo albums

Each centre should own a camera to record events and outings. Photo-graphs can then be displayed or arranged into albums for residents to peruse. It is also fun to record some events with slides, so that a follow-up activity can be to remember the event together, large as life, on the big screen.

Reading

Many people will take pleasure in listening to someone read to them. It is not always possible to judge how much a person is able to absorb but it may be enough to know there is someone there, talking to them in a gentle voice. Be careful to note whether such contact seems to relax or irritate the person as this will help you to judge if it is appropriate. Reading material can include poetry, ballads, short stories, selected newspaper articles, special interest books on topics known to be of interest to the resident, pictorial books and religious material. A volunteer, visitor or staff member will find it easier to spend time with the very frail person if they feel they can focus their attention on simple tasks such as reading.

Special afternoon teas and dinners

Too often frail older people are given a cup of tea or coffee in plastic feeder cups. Invariably some will spill and dribble much of the drink. Staff in nursing homes often report their amazement at the care that the same person takes when given a cup of tea in a nice china cup at a table decorated with tablecloth and flowers. Often the person will even manage to eat scones with jam and cream without mess. They will also enjoy the drink far more. I hate drinking coffee from a plastic cup on the rare occasions when it is necessary — it never tastes the same — but many people are forced to do so with every drink. There is always much appreciation expressed when it is offered in an attractive cup. It is also important to give people the opportunity to enjoy a special dinner in an attractive setting. For some it may be necessary to set the table in their room or other quiet place.

Taking time to chat

Sometimes activity workers and nursing staff are told to record the time spent talking with residents as 'reminiscence', 'reflective discussion' or 'individual socialisation'. There appears to be a need to justify and professionalise the benefits of sitting down to have a good old chat with a resident. In the interests of space and time, it should be enough to record that a chat has taken place, as it is one of the most important activities which staff can offer residents. Taking the time to chat will demonstrate that you enjoy and value that person's company. Chatting is something that most of us do many times a day. The frail older person will enjoy hearing about the things that are happening at the home, the little mishaps and amusing anecdotes. They may like to hear about your weekend or holiday or how your children are going at school. It will also be the time to find out how the resident is feeling and discover more about the background and interests of that person. These things are what human experience is all about. It may seem to be stating the obvious to add this here, but the technical phrases which are listed above suggest that sometimes this may be necessary.

Other activities

Once you have a clear picture of the frail resident's past interests you may find that an activity can be adapted to enable the person to participate (see Chapter 18). It may be that looking through books, watching films, videos, slides or a demonstration of an activity, or simply passively joining the group, is all that is needed to help the person retain their interest in a past skill or hobby. Taking the time to consider a person's interests and to develop a brief individual plan can make a great difference to the variety of activities which you offer frail residents. Some sample plans are listed at the end of Chapter 17.

Conclusion

The above activities offer a wide choice to the residents of aged care facilities. It is not an exhaustive list, but includes ideas which have been tested and have proved themselves popular. The format described provides a good base for trying out new ideas as they come to mind. The residents' committee, a socialisation assessment (see Chapter 17) and many informal chats will ensure that the selection of activities offered meets the various interests of the participants.

References

1. Rickard P. *Popular Activities and Games for Blind, Visually Impaired and Disabled People*. Published in 1986 by the Association for the Blind, 7 Mair Street Brighton Beach, Victoria 3186.
2. Dean E. *Esther Dean's Gardening Book: Growing without Digging*. Harper and Row (Australasia), 1981.
3. *The Ulverscroft Large Print Song Book*. Ulverscroft Large Print Books Ltd, Leicester, UK.
4. Price Bob. *Family Memories*. State Library of NSW, Australia, 1992.

Chapter 5
Special Events
*with Simone Keogh**

January 26, and the culmination of much anticipation and preparation is here at last. The January program committee had been in good form. The domestic supervisor had a friend who had won titles for shearing sheep. She was sure he would bring in half a dozen sheep to shear in the lounge. One of the nurses had a friend who'd probably love to spin the wool after it had been thrown across one of the tables and bundled. The usual barbecue lunch, damper, lamingtons and cans of beer were already on order. A few gum tree branches, yellow and green streamers and plenty of flies also helped denote the day.

The faithful band has arrived, complete with tea-chest bass and lagerphone; our bowling club band never ceases to amaze us with their generosity and creativity. The lagerphone player is a new recruit, 10 years old. For most of the staff, shorts and T-shirts predominate but a few are sporting the new national colours of green and gold, as are two of the babies who've decided to join today's event.

It's bush dancing, ballad reading, picnic races, joke telling and plenty of drinking for today's activities. It seems that almost everyone has chosen to stay in the lounge today. Fortunately the sheep are well behaved, and since she organised it, the domestic supervisor can't complain about the mess this time!

The importance of special events

This chapter will focus on special events, occasions which occur throughout the calendar year which can be celebrated with the residents of the home. All societies have celebrations of some kind. These events mark the

---

* Simone Keogh, formerly an activity coordinator at South Port Community Nursing Home, contributed the section on 'Cooking up a cruise'. She had successfully orchestrated a cruise with a little help from contacts in a nursing home in United States which had been running cruises for a number of years.

time of year, the seasons, and historical events worthy of remembrance. They offer participants time to ponder the past events and memories that the celebrations evoke, to look forward to the pleasure of the celebration itself, and share with others in the joy of the occasion.

Most social groups of people in the community create opportunities to get together and celebrate life with each other, and the residents of an extended care facility also have this need for celebration. Guests are a normal feature of a party, so an invitation should be extended to friends and relatives. These events help relatives and friends to take pleasure in their visits and provide a safe structure in which to relax and really enjoy each other's company.

Remember to use the residents' committee (see Chapter 2) to direct the frequency and nature of the events.

National days are particularly relevant if you have residents of that nationality in your home. We celebrated Greek national day because of one Greek resident and it was a great opportunity to give special attention to this man. He gained pleasure from seeing others participate in something of his culture, and enjoyed especially the homemade retsina donated by one of the kitchen staff. He didn't seem to mind that few others did! Fortunately, we had Greek staff in the kitchen and nursing departments and their advice and assistance were invaluable.

Another setting may have staff and residents from other cultural backgrounds. They will bring a whole new source of events to celebrate and many new ways to commemorate them. The ideas listed here will act as prompts from which the organisers can develop their own celebrations, tailor-made to the population of each centre.

You may start by celebrating the regular events of your country but do begin to introduce the national days and festivals of other countries. Be sure to celebrate every nation that is represented in your resident group and also introduce celebrations from cultures outside the experiences of your residents. This will add a far greater range of interesting activities, foods and music to the program. It is a terrific opportunity for people to discover more about other cultures and to celebrate and value people's differences.

Not all events need to be 'whiz-bang' occasions. A meal or afternoon tea and a few songs may be all that is needed for some occasions.

Special events are terrific for directing the regular program, as they create a whole new series of activities in preparation for the event. They provide the chance to cook, make, create, decorate, plan, talk about and anticipate the coming event, and are an excellent opportunity to involve the broader community in the fun. They also provide many chances to discover new talents among residents, staff and the local community; a whole new resource will be created.

They are also great morale boosters for both staff and residents.

Everyone can have fun and contribute significantly to the events and, as a result, enjoy their work more. This will rub off onto the quality of care which residents receive; they will find their staff friendlier and happier. I have found that the staff begin to see their work as far more than just a job; it becomes an occupation in which they care for and make lasting friends with the people in residence. Everyone benefits.

For each event, the many preparations will be structured similarly to those for the weekly activities listed in Chapter 4.

General requirements

Staff: Where possible all staff contribute to the day's fun in some way. This may be by dressing in appropriate costume, joining in the singing, dancing and competitions, or helping to involve the residents in the fun. Staff often volunteer their services because of a special talent or resource they have which is particularly appropriate to the day.

The program committee (see Chapter 2) plays an important role in planning and organising the many tasks required for each event. The brainstorming and the broad resource of contacts which come from this group will provide an inestimable supply of great ideas and people to contribute to the fun of the event. It ensures that everyone is prepared for the special demands that the event will place on each department. No department will complain of extra work if the staff have thought of the activity themselves!

It is worth noting that the convenor of this group may need special skills to enthuse and involve those staff who may be less than enthusiastic about joining in.

It is usually then the task of the activity coordinator to organise the preparations and entertainment, discuss foods with the kitchen, advertise the event, and oversee the activities on the day. If this person's hours of employment are limited, the various tasks can be delegated between nursing, domestic, kitchen and administrative staff.

Volunteers can be involved in all areas of the event, by contributing ideas, chasing up entertainers, and helping the residents to make costumes, food and decorations. They may provide the entertainment, or join in the dancing and singing. They are vital to the success of a busy celebratory day's activities (see Chapter 10).

Relatives are invited to attend, usually with a request to bring food and drink. They, too, are invited to wear appropriate costume and to contribute in similar ways to the volunteers.

Preparations provide residents with many tasks such as cooking special foods, and making decorations, costumes, prizes and advertising material.

The regular weekly activity program can focus on the event to direct the selection of activities within each group (see Chapter 4 for how to run the various group preparation activities). The local library can be a good resource for books (folklore is particularly useful), music and displays.

Entertainment may include a competition, some comical diversions and, where possible, appropriate musical entertainment. If you can, find some musicians from a local club who will provide, on a regular basis, music appropriate to the day.

Food: A party lunch or afternoon tea is most popular. This can be held in three ways: in the dining room, sitting as usual, with special food appropriate to the nationality of the day; finger food in the lounge; or a special afternoon tea. Where possible, involve the residents in preparing the food. Close communication with kitchen staff is necessary to make sure the special meal is convenient. Relatives and friends should also be invited to bring food.

Drinks: In addition to tea and coffee, an extra order of beer and soft drinks is needed; the bar then stays open throughout the party. Sherry and wine are also popular. Some fundraising may be needed for the extra supplies (see Chapter 3). Drinkers with more expensive tastes usually supply their own. The local supplier may like to donate a case of champagne occasionally, and staff and relatives also contribute. Volunteers and staff distribute the drinks.

Decorations can include flags, streamers, murals, table decorations and displays. It is particularly popular to invite children to work with the residents in creating these displays. Murals, displays and posters can surround the room — tourist bureaus and libraries are often good sources for posters. Staff and friends will usually bring in special items to create real-life displays.

Costumes: It is worth adding a little more atmosphere to the event by encouraging some people, particularly staff, to dress up for the occasion. Costumes become a great focus for conversation and joking, and my experience has been that dressing up also gives people permission to relax and have fun. Costumes can simply be funny hats, or complete outfits, any clothing that depicts the national colours and styles appropriate to the day. Residents should be free to decide if they will wear a costume; staff are encouraged more strongly!

Cost: Most of the events cost very little. Everyone contributes items from home. Staff and friends bring in extra food and drink. The party food which replaces the lunch or evening meal usually costs no more than the standard meal. Some fundraising or donations may be required to supplement the beverage supplies. Streamers and crêpe paper may need to be purchased but these can often be saved for later events and reused.

Choosing your celebrations and festivals

Most of the ideas that are suggested here have been collected by talking to people from various cultures. You can also look through the many books which are available about festivals and holidays. Talking to people is often more useful, however, as you gain a different perspective on the events and you may be able to draw upon resources from that person or their contacts.

Indigenous cultures

Be sure to also consider the indigenous cultures of your country, such as Aborigines or American Indians. Make contact with the local group in your area as they may have very different events and traditions to those of another area. They may be prepared to exhibit their dances and artefacts or offer guidance about suitable ways to celebrate their culture within your centre.

Whatever you do, do not restrict yourself to the events that are listed here. They reflect only a smattering of the range of cultures which are represented in our community. Use the format here as your guide then branch out into new countries and cultures wherever possible. Some dates have been added for your information, but space prevents listing full details for every event. A little homework will help you to discover the best ways to celebrate these events.

Religious festivals

Some general information is also interspersed about cultural events which relate to religious festivals. Some of these festivals are only relevant to the people of that religion. While it is important to be aware of the events so as to recognise the spiritual needs of individual residents, it may be more appropriate to connect the older person with her own cultural group to ensure that her religious and cultural needs are met. Care should be taken not to offend various cultural groups by trivialising deep spiritual rituals with a western, party version of the dates. It may be best to invite members of the local religious community to plan and provide entertainment and food which they feel it is appropriate to share with others. Other National Days can be added as appropriate. There are of course many more than those listed here but I had to stop somewhere! Design your own events around the formats suggested in this chapter.

YEARLY CALENDAR

January

1   New Year's Day
26   Australia Day
     Chinese New Year

February

14   St Valentines Day
     Holi — Hindu

March

1   St David's Day. Italian National
     Day
3   Festival of Dolls — Japan
     Shrove Tuesday: Pancake Day
17   St Patrick's Day
25   Greek National Day

April

     Easter
     Vesak — Buddhism
     St George's Day

May

5   Children's Day — Japan
     Mother's Day

June

     Queen's Birthday
25   St Paul's Day — Southern Italy

July

4   American Independence Day
14   Bastille Day

August

Whole month: Festival of the Hungry
Ghost
15   St Mary's Day — Malta
18   St Helena's Day — Malta

September

     Father's Day
     Show Day
     Grand Final Day
     Oktoberfest
18   St Joseph's Day — Southern
     Italy

October

     Spring Racing Carnival

November

1   Halloween
     Melbourne Cup Day
11   St Martin's Day. Dutch Name
     Day
4th Thursday: Thanksgiving
30   St Andrew's Day

December

25   Christmas Day
31   New Year's Eve

Spanish Fiestas
Other Religious Festivals
     Ramadan — Moslem
     Jewish Holidays

Other Ideas
     Annual Fete
     Birthday Parties: Residents
     Revue
     Sporting Events
     Holiday Cruise
     Guest Performers

The events

New Year's Day

After a heavy night, celebrating New Years's Day usually consists of sleeping in and recovery.

Australia Day: 26 January

Costume suggestions: Convicts, colonial, Aboriginal, ocker, sporting, bushy, green and gold, Ned Kelly, farmer, Australian animals.

Displays may include a campfire, cricket stumps, football jumpers and balls, green and gold streamers and the Australian flag.

Food: The great Australian barbecue, damper, billy tea, pies, pasties, lamingtons, pavlova, ice-creams . . . all are popular.

Drinks: Cans of light beer.

Entertainment: Ballads, a bush band, a classic Australian film such as *Man from Snowy River, Phar Lap, Gallipoli*, or the Dad and Dave films. These can be ordered from many film distributors (see Appendix C).

Activity ideas: Organise some bush picnic races, for example, egg and spoon, 3-legged, and sack races. Volunteers, staff and children can enter more difficult races with residents cheering them on. Sheep-shearing: invite

Laundry skips make for great sack races at bush picnics. Volunteers, staff and children race to the finishing line while residents cheer them on.

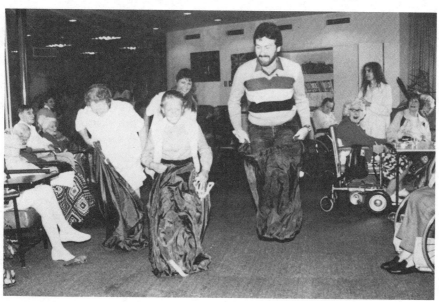

a shearer to bring in some sheep and a shearing stand and give a demonstration. Find someone to spin the wool as it comes off the sheep's back. This will create great interest for everyone.

Cars: Get a Holden car enthusiast to bring in an old car.

Aboriginal history: Display Aboriginal art and play their music, taste their food, or read some dreamtime legends.

Preparation activities: Make costumes, paint flags, make lamingtons, help make salads, butter rolls.

Staff contribution: Ask staff to bring pictures, costumes and other typically Australian objects to add to the atmosphere. Cooperation with kitchen staff is necessary to prepare them for the change in menu. All staff help to distribute the food.

Cost: Purchases may include square slab sponge cake for lamingtons, and green and gold crêpe paper for streamers. Allow for extra beer and soft drinks. Seek donations where possible.

I had never really celebrated Australia Day before working in a nursing home. I enjoyed the opportunity to do so, and I'm sure my feelings were shared by all those who attended the event.

Chinese New Year

This is a major time of celebration for most Asian countries. The date varies from year to year around the lunar calendar. It is a time of new beginnings. The old year is finished; everyone pays their debts, springcleans their home and buys new clothes in preparation for the holiday. It is a time for the family. In China it is their only real holiday. Everything closes for from three days to two weeks. The first day is spent at home with the family, feasting. The second day is spent visiting close relatives, and then later work associates and friends.

Children receive red packets of lucky money from visitors. Money is always given in even denominations as it is bad luck to be given anything in odd amounts. Similarly, oranges or mandarins are given out in even numbers.

Ancestral worship may occur at this time, and the household god is appeased before he leaves to return to the spirit world, so that he will take a good report with him. Fire crackers are set off to ward off evil spirits. After the three days when everything is made new and family obligations have been met, there is time for relaxation and gambling, usually in the form of mah-jong.

From these practices, a wide range of activities can be adapted in planning this event.

Attire: Coolie hats, kimonos, Chinese pyjamas. In western cultures most Chinese people now wear modern clothes at the time of the festival rather than adopting traditional dress.

Decorations: Collect posters from Asian travel agencies. Borrow a Chinese dragon from the Chinese community (if you celebrate late or early), or design and make your own displays with the help of school students.

Food: Chinese banquet, fortune cookies.

Music: Tapes of Chinese music, or live entertainment if possible.

Entertainment ideas: Invite a dragon to perform its dance. Have a Chinese cooking demonstration.

Activity ideas: Look at some Chinese legends and folklore; cook lunch together; go on outings to Chinatown and festivals.

Preparation activities: Displays and costume design; cooking.

Staff contribution: Assist with displays and costumes; all available staff distribute food at the mealtime.

Cost: The meal may actually cost less than the average meal, and be more nutritious. It is a good chance to test this style of cooking on residents for future inclusion in the normal menu.

There will be many things happening in the local community at the time of Chinese New Year which can provide opportunities for outings, activities and eating. It is a particularly valuable source of new and exciting experiences. Each individual will respond differently: some will hate the food, while others will love it, yet everyone will gain an up-to-date view of our multicultural society.

Hindu festivals

There are many Hindu festivals in India. One is Holi, which is a five-day celebration of the arrival of spring flowers in late February. It represents the love of the god Krishna for a girl called Radha. It is the festival of colour — everyone wears bright clothing and people buy red powder and coloured water to throw over each other. They have processions, dancing, feasting and bonfires to burn images of demons, and they carry statues of the gods around the streets on floats.

St Valentine's Day: 14 February

We all need a little romance in our lives and older people are not exempt from this need. Most of us gain some pleasure from dressing up and dining in style. In addition, we are all in need of a little care and attention, and this day provides on excuse to cuddle and touch those we care about. Sometimes the extended care setting tends to restrict opportunities to express these needs. This event can help to create a safe atmosphere to encourage more chances for caring, touching, and expressions of warmth and friendship between staff, residents and relatives.

Attire: Evening wear, tails, bow tie, frilly, flouncy, pastel attire, with pink the predominant colour.

Decorations: Pink hearts, paper and fresh flowers, pink and white streamers, doves, cupids, candles.

Food: A candlelit dinner party, with the dining room decorated to look like a restaurant; tables decorated with flowers, candles and chocolates. Design a special menu, a three-course meal with all the trimmings. Display the menu on a blackboard or large decorated sign. Available staff welcome residents to the café and show them to their tables with special flair. A roving musician can serenade everyone during the meal.

Entertainment ideas: Show a classic romantic film, for example, a Fred Astaire and Ginger Rogers movie, or one with Gene Kelly or Judy Garland (see Appendix C). Invite an entertainer(s) to play romantic music. Suitable background music could also be played throughout the day to create a romantic atmosphere.

Activity ideas: Send a Valentine's card from the women to the men and/or vice versa, write poetry, love letters. Arrange for some residents and staff to rehearse songs to serenade other residents and staff. Have ballroom dancing, in wheelchairs if necessary.

Preparation activities: Make paper hearts and Valentine cards, rehearse any of the above activities, make chocolates, cream puffs and ice-cream (find someone with a churn).

Staff contribution: More time than usual should be allowed for residents to eat their meal. Where possible, activity, therapy and nursing staff should help the domestic staff to serve the meals. Staff may like to contribute to musical items and join in the dancing and singing.

Cost: Where possible, ingredients for cooking are obtained through the kitchen supplies. You may need to allow extra funds for special ingredients.

St David's Day: 1 March

This is the Welsh national day so leeks should dominate the menu. Not all events need to be major — this activity could simply centre on lunch.

Dress: The dress for the day could be coal-mining attire.

Activity ideas: Sing hymns and classical songs.

Italian National Day: 1 March

Celebrate with red, green and white flags, Italian music or entertainers, much spaghetti, pizza and antipasto, garlic bread, vino, grape crushing, dancing and singing.

Other Italian Celebrations

Most towns throughout Southern Italy will have their own Saint for whom they set aside a holiday. For example in Copetino near Lecce, St Joseph's Day is celebrated on 18 September. The celebrations begin on the 16th with feasts, carnivals, outdoor opera, parades, stalls of sweets and ice-creams. Everyone wears new clothes and eats specially prepared meat balls made of donkey or horse meat along with much pasta and wine. In the nearby town of Galatina, St Paul's Day is celebrated on 25 June. In that town there is a well full of snakes and it is believed that if you drink the water from this well you will be healed of afflictions. Similar festivities occur in other towns throughout Italy. Other European countries, such as Malta, also have various Saint's Days to celebrate. Be sure to find out the Saint's Days of your residents and research ways to celebrate them if you can.

Japan — Festival of Dolls: 3 March

Collect as many different dolls from around the world as possible, and work with a local school to make displays. Residents may wish to decorate and dress dolls in different clothing. Make it a children's day, inviting the children of relatives, staff and local schools. Have competitions and face painting, with games and party food. Get the children and residents to make paper lanterns together. Decorate the centre and invite dancers and entertainers. Eat Japanese food.

Shrove Tuesday

Shrove Tuesday is pancake day, when pancakes are made before the beginning of Lent in the build-up to Easter. It marks the beginning of a period when some people choose to go without luxuries to prepare themselves for the Easter Passion. One need not go without luxuries to find an excuse to make and eat pancakes.

Activities: Cook and eat pancakes, or have pancake-tossing competitions and races.

St Patrick's Day: 17 March

Costumes: As much green as possible, with shamrocks wherever you can pin them.

Decorations: Green streamers, leprechauns, shamrocks. Invite the local primary school to help with decorations and displays, and to join the residents in making a collage rainbow, with a pot of gold at its base. A joke sheet can be displayed, requesting contributions.

Food: Potatoes should dominate the menu; an Irish stew with heaps of mashed potato, followed by an oatmeal dessert, would be suitable.

Alternatively, party food in the lounge would suffice, to create a party atmosphere.

Drink: Apart from the usual beer and soft drink, Irish whisky is also needed.

Entertainment ideas: Irish folk singing and dancing are always lots of fun. There are many good Irish entertainers about who are usually happy to donate some of their time to entertain residents. However, if St Patrick's Day falls at the weekend, change the date, as all the Irish entertainers will be in the city celebrating!

Activity ideas: Joke telling, ballads and yarns are all fun.

Preparation activities: Make the rainbow mural and shamrock ribbons. Paint the flag, shamrock displays and leprechauns. Bake Irish biscuits and cakes, cook anything with potatoes.

Staff contribution: Bring anything green, tell jokes, join in an Irish jig or two.

Cost: Irish whisky.

Greek National Day: 25 March/28 October

There are two dates for celebrating Greek National Day so choose the one that best suits your program.

Costume: Greek national costume, peasant dress, military, or traditional styles.

Everyone, including our one Greek resident, enjoys the dancing troop on Greek National day.

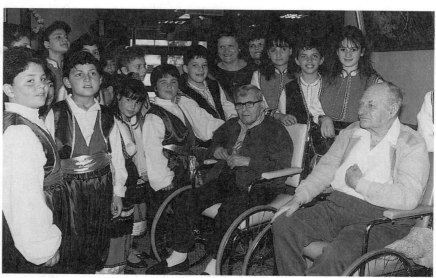

Displays: The Greek flag, blue and white streamers, grapes, basket-woven bottles and crusty bread will help set the scene.

Food: If you are fortunate enough to have Greek staff helping in the kitchen, as we did, they may be able to provide a spit to roast a lamb for lunch. In our case, they also made Greek dips and salads, and included olives, fetta cheese and crusty bread in the menu, followed by baklava for dessert, made by the residents.

Drink: Include a small amount of retsina (Greek wine) and ouzo in the drink supply, although only Greek residents tend to drink this with relish. The usual extra requirement of beer and soft drinks is also necessary.

Entertainment ideas: A local high school may have a Greek dancing group, which can perform Greek dancing and teach staff and friends the basics. Ask the Greek Orthodox Community to help you find a dancing group. If the sun shines, all the eating and activity can take place outside on the lawn. This is a particularly successful event, and a great opportunity to focus attention on Greek residents.

Staff contribution: This activity places an extra load on the kitchen, although residents can do much of the work, preparing the simpler salads,

One of the kitchen staff who is Greek brings along a spit for the occasion.

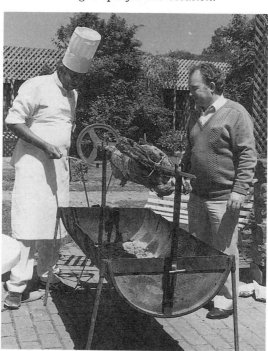

bread, dips and the Greek desserts. The cook will need to supervise the spit, but he/she is likely to enjoy a change of scenery. In our setting, the Greek kitchen assistants took a special interest in the preparations, supervised the purchase of ingredients and provided many special touches, such as homemade wine, salads and dips.

The staff in your kitchen may be able to cook other national specialties that can be presented on the appropriate national day.

Activity ideas: The day centres on lunch. Dancing follows soon after, so all available staff participate in the lunch distribution and eating, followed by a time for dancing together.

Cost: The lamb is purchased through kitchen supplies; staff pay for their lunch. If a spit is not available, one can be hired commercially, which does add significantly to the cost of the meal. It may be possible to make one with a little ingenuity on someone's part.

Easter

Easter is many different things to different people. Find out what your residents would most like to focus on. For example, with a Christian focus, you may organise special services and provide an opportunity for residents to attend their local church, or see a passion play or the *Messiah*. It is also a spring festival in the northern hemisphere, hence the Easter eggs and bunnies. For others it is a time for a major sporting event, such as the Stawell Gift foot race, so activities can centre on these events.

Activity ideas: A large Easter rabbit display can be created with the help of school children. Egg-dying; chocolate-making; reminiscing groups about Easter in the past and how it has changed. A debate: 'Should Easter be so commercialised?' Activities can incorporate looking at how Easter is celebrated in other countries, for example, the Spring Festivals, Passion plays, cooking special Easter foods from other countries. On Easter Sunday, a staff member may like to dress as the Easter bunny to distribute Easter eggs to the residents.

Cost: Purchase of eggs.

Vesak — Buddhism: April–May

Vesak celebrates the life of Buddha. Buddhists gather at the temple and decorate the statues with flowers and listen to Buddha's teachings. Homes are decorated with flowers and candles and presents are given. Captured birds are set free, and gifts are left for the poor.

St George's Day: 23 April

This day could focus on the British royal family and anything which reminds residents of the 'home' country. This event could be celebrated in conjunction with the Queen's Birthday.

Costumes: Royalty, button suits, country gentry, cockney, historical.

Decorations: Union Jacks, pictures of royalty and English scenery.

Food: Devonshire tea, or a particularly English lunch such as beef Wellington, cornish pasties, pork pies, or roast beef and Yorkshire pudding. Many residents may have a particular food which, for them, conjures up thoughts of England. Cook these where possible.

Activity ideas: Cookery, discussions about the royal family, look at books, show a video about the royal family or England. Sing old English songs or read some English stories. Show a classic English movie such as *Oliver Twist*, *Great Expectations*, *Wuthering Heights*, *Rebecca* or *Jane Eyre*.

Mother's Day: 2nd Sunday in May

The best way to celebrate Mother's Day is to have a special afternoon tea on the day. An elaborate cake could be made, together with other afternoon tea specialties. Single chrysanthemums can be pinned to everyone: residents, staff and friends.

Preparation activities: The local school children may like to make flowers and cards for the ladies. Homemade chocolates would also go down well.

It should also be a special family day; many relatives will visit anyway but others may need to be encouraged to come and join in the afternoon tea. Send everyone a special invitation card. Some relatives may like to contribute cakes for the occasion. As it is Sunday, with some limits on staff, it is usually enough to celebrate the day with afternoon tea and the chance for visitors to chat to their relatives. Some musical entertainment may be appropriate.

Cost: Purchase of flowers; cards can be homemade.

Queen's Birthday: 1st Monday in June

This is another occasion for a special afternoon tea with particularly English delicacies made by the residents. Special tablecloths, china, silverware and serviettes will help to set the atmosphere for a really high-class event. One of the residents may like to dress as the Queen Mother and give the birthday message.

Activity ideas: Of course, 'God Save the Queen' should be sung a number of times. See St George's Day for further ideas.

Staff contribution: Whoever is available may like to help by supplying the special touches and contributing to the atmosphere of the social occasion.

American Independence Day: 4 July

Costume suggestions: Cowboys and Indians, cabaret girls, gangsters, gridiron players, cheerleaders, supermen and women, Country and Western characters, red, white and blue everything, Uncle Sam, cavalry, Abraham Lincoln, Statue of Liberty, pin-up girls.

Displays: Decorate the walls with the American flag, red, white and blue streamers, and pictures of the Wild West, hamburgers and hot dogs. Set the room up to look like a saloon bar.

Food: Fried chicken, hamburgers, hot dogs, chips, pumpkin pie, blueberry and apple pie. A party lunch in the lounge works best for these occasions.

Entertainment ideas: Items could include Country and Western singing, bathing beauty competitions or 'Guess the Legs', cabaret saloon-bar style entertainment, or a barber shop quartet. Show an American film, particularly an MGM great (see 'Films' in Chapter 4 for details).

Preparation activities: Make Uncle Sam hats, bake pumpkin, apple and blueberry pies, make food poster displays, paint the flag and prepare costumes. Crumb the chicken pieces for the cook.

Staff contribution: Dress up and join in the fun; stage a shoot-out; attempt an abduction of a resident; hand out the food and drinks; and join in the competitions and singing.

Cost: Allow extra funds for crêpe paper for streamers.

Bastille Day: 14 July

As Bastille Day follows closely behind 4 July, you may like to limit this to an afternoon event. However, if you feel like further reducing the winter doldrums, go the whole hog! Make sure the streamers from 4 July stay up for this date.

Costumes: Red, white and blue again, hats and bonnets, berets, a French artist, cabaret girls, slinky high-heeled fashions, striped T-shirts are all appropriate.

Displays: Cover the walls with French paintings, flags, streamers, and a picture of the Eiffel tower. Create a French café with checkered tablecloths, waitresses in tiny aprons and black skirts, and a roving musician.

Food: If a luncheon, serve a café-style meal in the dining room, with hors d'oeuvres, pâté, vichyssoise, quiche lorraine, crêpes, French pastries. For an afternoon tea celebration serve French pastries, cheese, hors d'oeuvres.

Drink: Red and white wine should be served where appropriate to the meal.

Entertainment ideas: Play Edith Piaf or Maurice Chevalier as background music, and have a roving musician at lunch. Give a fashion parade, invite residents and staff to wear their classiest outfits for the parade.

Preparation activities: Cook!

Staff contribution: A luncheon such as this takes a lot of effort. Despite the fact that the residents cook all the food, the domestic staff need extra assistance to serve and supervise such an extensive meal.

Cost: Although the food sounds expensive, quantities need only be small; and, as the food is prepared by residents and consists mainly of vegetable dishes, it will cost no more than a standard more meat-oriented meal.

Moon Cake Festival — Festival of the Hungry Ghost: August

Throughout August Chinese people enter into a range of activities to ward off ghosts for the year and to ensure that their ancestors have a safe and comfortable passage to heaven. Moon Cakes are cooked during this time. Traditional foods are cooked and set beside the road for spirits to consume. In the morning it is claimed that the food has lost its flavour because the spirits have fed from it. A range of activities are engaged in to ward off spirits, such as burning joss sticks and feeding the spirits to send them away for another year. Children are not allowed to go swimming or to go out at night because of lurking ghosts. Communities gather and build elaborate temporary structures to perform outdoor operas.

Ancestors are assisted with their assent to heaven by burning gold paper money, paper cars, paper houses, and other material objects to ensure that their souls will know comfort in heaven. These paper effigies are often very detailed and beautiful. A range of visiting exhibitions, demonstrations and performances could occur in August to acknowledge this time.

Father's Day — see Mother's Day

Show Day

If you are brave you can take a small group of residents to the show. Or bring the show home so that everyone can enjoy the animals, show bags, competitions and side shows together.

Costumes: Farmer Brown, country bumpkin, horse riders, clowns, animals and spectators.

Displays: Side shows, animal displays, streamers, advertising posters, show bags, a spinning wheel.

Activities on the day

DOG SHOW: Invite staff, relatives and volunteers to bring in their pets. If you know an animal judge, all the better; otherwise choose someone with a sense of humour.

BABY SHOW: Invite anyone who has a baby to enter it, and anyone who is prepared to dress (and act) like a baby to enter too.

SIDE EVENTS: Borrow a spinning wheel from a local club. Play lucky quoits — throw the quoits onto a prize to win it, for example, beer, champagne, soft drink. Include coin-throwing competitions. Set up a small animal display with rabbits, guinea pigs, budgies, chickens and lambs — anything that will add to the atmosphere of a showground.

Food: A party lunch in the lounge, with finger food, is best for these occasions. Junk food should predominate, such as crisps, twisties, hot dogs, hamburgers, party pies, sausage rolls, etc. Ice-cream cones are fine for dessert.

Preparation activities

SHOW BAGS: Approach local businesses to donate items for the show bags. They can include biscuits, after-dinner mints, cheese sticks, novelty jams, party hats, streamers and small gifts. In addition, make gingerbread men, homemade sweets and shortbread to add to the bags. The packaging and bagging of all these items provides much activity prior to the day.

BABY AND DOG SHOW SASHES: Make sashes depicting winning categories, both humorous and serious, for example, the cutest, brightest, hairiest, cleverest and most original!

Staff contribution: As this will be a busy day, all staff are asked to take part, wherever possible, by dressing up, bringing in babies, dogs and other pets, and helping with lunch distribution.

Cost: Allow extra funds for party hats, streamers and prizes.

Oktoberfest

This is a two-week festival which ends on the first Sunday in October. It originally celebrated the marriage of the first king of Bavaria in 1810, but now celebrates the Oktoberfest for its own sake. The beginning of the festival is marked by a parade of decorated brewery carts and pageants. It is followed by two weeks of parties, parades, fancy dress and sumptuous feasts.

Costumes: Bavarian national dress. Leather shorts and Bavarian hats, peasant clothes, fancy dress.

Displays: Bavarian posters, horses, beer posters, travel displays.

Food: Weisswurst, schaschlik, leberkas, kartoffelpuffer, sauerkraut, eisbein, kassler, ochs am spiess, backhandl, brezel, horse radish, struedel-kuchen and apfelstrudel.

Activity ideas: Much drinking of beer, singing and folk dancing, knee slapping.

Entertainment: Bavarian folk band or recorded music; folk dancing display.

Preparation activities: Outings with residents to shop for the various special foods at a continental deli or market.

Outing: Take a group of residents to the Oktoberfest celebrations held in your city.

Grand Final Day, Australian Rules Football

On the Saturday, the main activity will be, of course, to watch the match. Make sure lunch is served in the lounge while viewing the preliminary games and events. The meal should consist of pies and pasties, hot dogs and sausage rolls to add to the atmosphere. Beer, preferably in cans, should be available throughout the match.

The week before the game should set the scene for Saturday: decorate the lounge with the team colours; run football clinics; stage a football match of your own (see 'Games' in Chapter 4); run a football quiz, or a debate about the changing face of football over the years. An old football celebrity could be invited to visit. Keen football fans should be able to make regular trips to matches throughout the season.

Costumes: On the day, all staff should be dressed either as football players or spectators. Residents may also like to sport the team colours.

Spring racing carnivals

With spring, begin the racing carnivals which lead to the major racing cup for your city or town. Spring can be celebrated simply with flower displays, flower arrangement demonstrations and displays, or outings to local and botanical gardens. However, many people also enjoy the carnival atmosphere of the racing circuit and should have some chance to go to the races or at least place some bets during this time.

Caulfield cup (or local cup prior to the major racing event in your State)

This is the time to start building up for the major cup, for example, the Melbourne Cup. A trip to the races would be timely. The race should be screened on the day, and bets placed at the local TAB. The film *Phar Lap* could also be screened around this time to help set the scene for the major city cup. Invite an old jockey, trainer or racing commentator to visit. Reminiscing groups about races past and present will also add to a sense of anticipation. A sweep should be organised, preferably by one of the residents, in which everyone is free to participate.

Halloween: 31 October

The feast of All Saints, this is a time to ward of evil spirits and ghosts and to honour the saints of yesteryears.

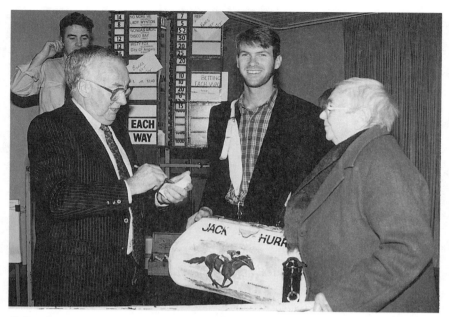

Collecting the winnings! Include a trip to the races as part of the racing carnival fever.

Costumes: Invite local children to dress as ghosts, witches, devils, monsters, ghouls, elves and fairies. Some staff and residents may wish to dress up too.

Displays: Turnips and pumpkins carved into faces with candles inside, a mural of Halloween characters, lanterns and ghosts everywhere.

Food: Party foods, soups and pumpkin pies to use up the insides of all the vegetable lanterns!

Activity ideas: Apple bobbing or apples on strings, trick or treat, hold a bonfire outside and tell stories, toast marshmallows, roast potatoes and apples. A few days later, residents can help the gardener to spread the ashes of the bonfire around the garden. This is a traditional part of Halloween designed to magically bring about a good crop.

Preparation activities: Work with a local school to make displays, carve vegetables and make lollies and truffles for trick or treat.

Melbourne Cup Day: early November

This can be the biggest event of the year apart from Christmas and, if celebrated to the full, the centre can be the most exciting place to be on Cup Day. The car park or even the stand at the racetrack can't match the fun. As it is a public holiday (in Victoria), all relatives, friends, volunteers,

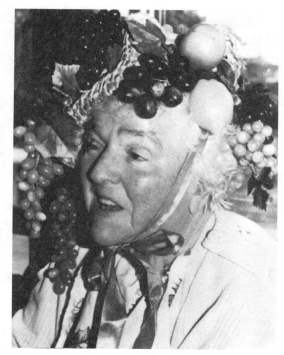

*Carmen Miranda has her family to thank for
her prize-winning head attire.*

staff and their families are invited to attend. The major focus of the day
is of course the race itself, but other activities include a fashion parade,
the hat competition, your own Wheelchair Cup, the sweep and as much
eating and drinking as possible!

Costumes: The crazier the better, or dress for the Fashions in the Field.
Entry to the premises requires the wearing of some form of head-dress.

Food: Party food is served in the lounge at lunchtime. It must include
chicken and champagne.

Drink: Extra supplies are necessary, but guests are invited to bring their
own. Your drink supplier may like to donate a crate of champagne for the
occasion.

Activity ideas: The day usually begins at 11am, with the hat judging;
a variety of categories provides for a number of winners. Throughout the
day the central focus is the bookmaker's table where bets are taken for all
the races and placed at the local TAB.

Stage the wheelchair race after lunch. About six residents volunteer to
take on the name of a cup horse, e.g. Quick as a Dash Jack, and they each
require a pusher. The course is set out along a corridor leading into the

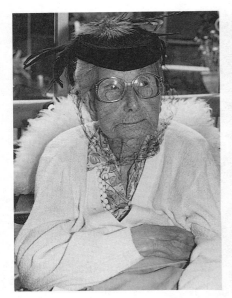 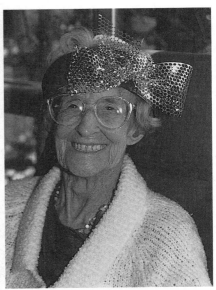

Others go for style rather than originality.

lounge. Lines about 1 metre apart are marked with masking tape along the course. A large die is thrown by each 'horse' who moves the given number of spaces forward. The first to cross the finishing line, with an exact throw of the die, wins. Places are then played for. A betting ring is also organised for this event.

Other activities include a fashion parade of costumes, and musical entertainment with singing and dancing. The day culminates with the viewing of the race.

Preparation activities: Hat creations need to be started a few weeks before the event. Relatives may like to assist their resident to create a hat which best reflects their personality and interests.

Other activities could include food preparation. Children can help residents to create a mural depicting the event. A collage of magazine photos along a race track is most effective. This can then be redisplayed in following years. One of the residents can organise the sweep during the week before the event.

Staff contribution: The activity organisers should work on this public holiday and take another day off in its stead. All staff who are not working should be encouraged to come with their families to celebrate the event. Everyone then participates in whatever way they prefer, placing bets, helping with food preparation and distribution, singing, dancing or wheelchair pushing. All come with some form of head attire and usually a costume to match. Staff and volunteers supply the musical entertainment.

Cost: The extra order of drinks will be the greatest cost, though staff and relatives are encouraged to bring their own. Prizes for competitions are also needed, and donations should be sought for these.

Thanksgiving: fourth Thursday in November

Thanksgiving is a time for being thankful for many blessings, particularly for the autumn harvests of the northern hemisphere. In the United States it marks the first harvests which the local Indians helped the Pilgrims to grow. Hence the turkey, sweet potatoes, corn and pumpkin. For some, the day will include a special thanksgiving church service, but everyone joins together with family and friends for a roast meal with these foods as its base.

Many residents may be encouraged to join their families at home on this day, others may wish to invite selected friends or relatives to join them for a thanksgiving luncheon at the centre.

Displays: A harvest theme; Pilgrim and American Indian displays of clothing, artefacts, posters from the United States.

Food: Roast turkey, cranberry sauce, sweet potato, roast pumpkin, corn and pumpkin pie.

Activity ideas: Centred around family get togethers, eating and recovery!

St Andrew's Day: 30 November

This is a very popular day to celebrate, as many people have some degree of Scottish heritage.

Costumes: Tartan!

Displays: Tartan, thistles, bagpipes, Highland pictures, the flag of the rampant lion.

Food: Oatmeal cookies for morning tea, haggis, Scottish bun and short-bread as part of the party lunch or afternoon tea.

Entertainment ideas: Invite a bagpipe player to pipe in the haggis. Bagpipe music will never fail to bring tears to the eyes of many residents. A Scottish volunteer may offer to help with the entertainment. A local Highland dancing group may like to demonstrate its skills.

Preparation activities: Make shortbread, Scottish bun, oatmeal cookies. Paint flags: blue with a white diagonal cross; a red rearing lion on a yellow background. Make the displays listed above.

Staff contribution: Help residents dress for the occasion, wear as much tartan as possible, and join in the fun.

Cost: Scottish whisky and haggis need to be purchased (if donations can't be obtained).

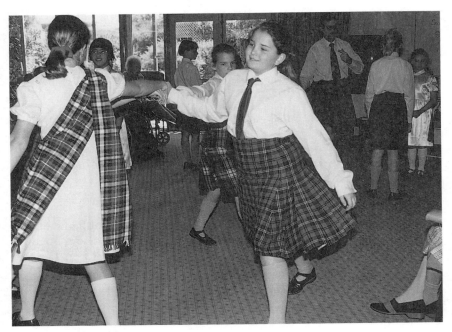

St Andrews Day is always very popular.

Christmas: 25 December

Christmas is a major event. The management committee needs to assign funds to buy gifts for residents, and for the food and decorations. Christmas belongs to the residents, so they should be encouraged to take part in as much of the preparation as possible. An institution can seem to do every-thing for the resident, taking control and placing residents in a position of care receipt only. In the normal home environment, everyone works together, so participation in the Christmas preparations helps to restore a sense of ownership and homeliness to the centre. Preparations begin in November, with cooking and the making of gifts and decorations.

Cooking starts in November with the Christmas puddings, which are then hung near the lounge area until Christmas Day. The Christmas cake (well soaked with brandy), shortbread, chocolate Christmas trees, White Christmas, homemade sweets and chocolates can all be prepared at various times before the day. You may find the men come to the fore at Christmas time and take over as chief pudding and cake cooks whereas, at other times of the year, they may rarely volunteer to join a cooking group.

Gift ideas: Residents make gifts to give to their key relative or friend. Choose quick, simple crafts so that the more able residents can make more than one gift and thus enable the very confused and disabled residents to give gifts too. Ideas include:

- pot pourri
- pomanders (oranges covered with cloves)
- lavender sachets
- pressed flower pictures
- potted plant cuttings
- dried flower arrangements
- homemade sweets
- miniature Christmas puddings
- shortbread
- bread dough decorations

Residents also like the opportunity to give something to staff, so packages of homemade sweets can be made to give to each staff member.

Christmas shopping: A number of shopping trips should be arranged so that all residents who would like to are able to buy gifts for their relatives. Afternoon tea at a café adds to the outing.

Decorations: Find out who are the most talented decorators among staff and volunteers. They can hang the purchased decorations, design and make the table decorations with residents, and organise residents to decorate the Christmas tree in the week before Christmas. Some decorations can be made easily by residents.

Bread dough decorations: A 2:1 mixture of flour and salt, with enough water to knead it into a dough, can be cut with biscuit cutters or modelled into shape. The shapes are baked in a slow oven, then painted with enamel paint and Estapol.

Choir boys/angels: These can be made by folding *Reader's Digest* magazines into a cone then spray painting red or gold; paper doilies, ping-pong balls and cardboard wings give finishing touches.

Pompoms can be decorated to look like snowmen, Santa Claus or Christmas baubles. Many craft books contain simple ideas for quick, attractive decorations.

Residents' gifts: Ask the nursing staff to make a list of gift ideas which suit the personality of each resident. A couple of nurses can then spend a morning shopping for them.

On the day: A volunteer dresses as Father Christmas and delivers gifts to everyone at breakfast time. Residents choose whether to have Christmas out with their families, or to invite a relative to join them for lunch. You may like to provide pre-dinner drinks and hors d'oeuvres for all relatives, friends, volunteers and other staff who would like to drop in.

Christmas marks a chance to look back over the year and say thank you to the residents, staff and volunteers for the special contributions they all make to the life of the centre. A full Christmas dinner is then served in the dining room.

New Year's Eve: 31 December

Most residents request a party to be held in the evening with musical entertainment and an open bar. The party should be based on the types of parties which occur in the larger community. Because many staff are away at this time of year, residents may like to organise the event themselves through the residents' committee.

Decorations: The decorations from Christmas should still be in place. This will be enough to mark the festive occasion.

Activity ideas: The daytime will be spent resting in preparation for the late night. Many residents will need an afternoon's nap to make it through the night. During the evening, card and table games, singalongs and musical entertainment can be arranged by the committee.

Entertainment: It is usually difficult to find outsiders who will entertain on New Year's Eve, so it is best to draw on the talents of the residents, the staff working the late shift, and the relatives and friends who wish to attend.

Food: Party food should be prepared ahead of time for the evening.

Drink: Extra supplies will certainly be required for this night. Some residents may prefer to provide their own drinks, so a special trip to the liquor store may be necessary to obtain each individual's order.

Cost: Residents meet the costs of the extra drinks. There's usually a good supply of drinks left over from Christmas, particularly if the donation system has worked well.

Spanish Speaking Countries

Most of the fiestas and holidays in Spain and other Spanish speaking countries are based around the Roman Catholic calendar. Each local area has its patron Saint for whom it holds celebrations, including fireworks, dancing, candlelit prayers, cockfights and bullfights. The streets are decorated with flowers and coloured tissue paper.

Spain

In Spain the week before Easter is Holy week which includes all of these festive activities and beauty contests. In July there is the Fiesta of San Fermin when bulls are let loose in the streets and young men run ahead of them to the bullfight ring.

Mexico

Independence Days are September 15 and 16, other Saint's Days are celebrated throughout the year. A major holiday is Guadalupe Day, which celebrates the appearance of the Virgin Guadalupe, as an Indian maiden, on 12 December in Mexico City. They also celebrate the nine days before Christmas, acting out the journey of Mary and Joseph to Bethlehem. Known as Pasoda, each night children take turns to hit a pinata with a stick while blindfolded. A pinata is an earthenware or papier-mâché animal filled with fruit, sweets and toys.

Any one of the Saint's Days or holidays could be selected as a date to celebrate. Or choose Mexico or Spain as the destination of holiday cruise (*Cooking up a cruise* p. 113).

Costumes: Bull fighters, bulls, dancers, peasant dress, national dress.

Food: Mexican food, or Spanish foods. Tortillas, nachos, dips, tacos, bean dishes etc.

Decorations: Flowers, colourful decorations, posters, displays of clothing, fabrics, pinatas.

Activity ideas: Break pinatas, hold a bullfight, have dancing and music, hold a beauty contest for men and women.

Entertainment ideas: Invite Spanish dancers from the local dancing school to demonstrate their skills. (We had a charge nurse who learnt Spanish dancing and performed for us.) Or invite a band to play. The music of many South American cultures is wonderful, both lively and lilting.

Preparation activities: Work with a local school to make pinatas and other decorations. Prepare many of the foods with residents.

Other Religious Festivals

Ramadan

Ramadan is a Moslem religious festival which varies from year to year as it follows the lunar calendar. This means it is celebrated ten days earlier each year. Ramadan is celebrated across Moslem communities in Africa, Pakistan and India, Arabic and Asian communities. For a month, no food, drink or cigarettes are consumed between sunrise and sunset. At sunset the fast is broken with a drink of water and three dates and then food is eaten before bed and again early before sunrise. During this time there are no parties or visiting. It is a time for self-discipline, prayer and restraint.

The fast is broken as the rim of a new moon appears over the horizon. This time is known as Id-Ul-Fitr, and consists of three days of partying and visiting. Children are given money and where possible everyone gets a new set of clothes. But it is also a time to give money to the poor. Each country has its own special foods which are cooked for Id. For example, in Pakistan it is foods such as lamb korma, dry mince dishes, biryani, a special beef curry known as nihari, chapattis, pakora and special desserts made with almonds, sultanas, vermicelli and rice. Pakistani people wear new clothes of Shalwar Quameez — long baggy pants with a long over-dress, and a scarf added for the women.

Two months and ten days later there is a time of sacrifice known as Id-Ul-Azahr. This follows the period which would be the end of a time of pilgrimage to Mecca. Groups of families and friends buy a sheep or cow, cook it and share it among themselves and the poor.

Jewish Holidays

There are many different holy days and events which the Jewish culture celebrate. They include Purim, Passover, Shavuot, Rosh Hashanah or Jewish New Year which ends with Yom Kippur, and Hanukkah. Each of these events relates to a significant event recorded in the Old Testament. Some include periods of fasting followed by special foods and celebrations which vary from country to country. Connect your Jewish residents with a local Jewish community so they can share in relevant events. Also, invite members of the community to bring in samples of their food, music, traditional dress, etc for other residents to experience.

Other Ideas

Winter ideas: Snowmen, ski displays, slides and films about winter. Hot spiced wines, thick soups, steamed puddings; hold Christmas in June in southern countries. Or fight the winter blues by recreating summer with an Hawaiian celebration, including leis, hula skirts, tropical foods and fruits and dancing.

Country and western day: Country music, clothing, farm animals, hay bales, home country cooking.

International Day: Invite staff and relatives to dress in the national clothing of their origins and to bring food from that country. The food can be shared over lunch with a variety of international musical performances throughout the afternoon. (See other theme ideas in Chapter 4 which can be used to mark a special day's activities.)

Annual fete

The annual fete can be a major source of funds for many of the activities and programs described. It may also be possible to fund part of the wage for the coordinator of volunteers with the proceeds, as a properly organised fete can raise over $5000. The fete is also a valuable event in itself as it provides a wonderful external motivator for a wide range of activities. Most people prefer to make things for a reason.

The ever-popular jams, chutneys, pickles and preserves can keep a cooking group at work all year round. It gives many residents the chance to cook all their old tried and true recipes again. Volunteers and residents can get together to make craft and novelty items to sell (see 'Craft and gift-making' in Chapter 4 p. 46). It also provides an opportunity for residents to assume responsibility for the sale of these items on the day.

The fete can be organised by an auxiliary, providing yet another area in which volunteers can be involved. Some volunteers much prefer fundraising to direct involvement in the centre's activities.

Fete committee: A committee comprising auxiliary, voluntary, administrative, nursing and activity staff, in addition to management committee representatives, will be needed if serious fundraising is to occur. Preparations will include special sideshows, the white elephant stall, Devonshire Tea, hire of equipment and musical entertainment.

Stalls: Many different stalls can be organised. The local community can contribute to cake, sweets, garden, white elephant, craft, secondhand books and clothing stalls. Someone's garage may be needed to collect items throughout the year. Residents can be involved in the collection and sales.

Residents' stall: In addition, it is worth having a special stall to which only residents contribute, so they can tally their own contribution to the final sum raised. This will help residents to feel they are significant contributors and give them some sense of ownership. Items can include jams, cakes, crafts, novelty items, plant cuttings and wooden toys.

Sideshows: Pony rides, merry-go-rounds, air castles, clowns, pie-throwing competitions, face painting, continental sausage and hot dog stall, fairy floss, personalised badge and computer poster-making all help to raise extra funds and add atmosphere.

Raffles: Local businesses can be approached to donate items for a large raffle. Other raffles can be ongoing throughout the year to add further funds; for example, a Christmas hamper raffle. The auxiliary is usually best equipped for this kind of work.

Licence: Obtain permission from the appropriate government bodies for the raffles and stalls.

Birthday parties

Residents' parties can take a number of forms. There may simply be a cake and a few songs for individuals on their particular birthday. If a few residents have birthdays close together, a larger, combined party may be arranged. If it is a particularly significant birthday, such as an 80th, 90th or 100th, a bigger party could be arranged. In any case, the families of these residents should be involved as much as possible. The resident can decide with them what sort of party he or she would like.

Centre parties: The birthday of your centre is another good excuse for a party — the celebrations can be similar to those described for special events.

Federal, State and council elections

Arrangements should be made for postal voting, or a voting booth can be set up by the electoral office at the home on the day of the election.

Revue

Every year or so, depending on the energy of the organisers, an evening revue can be performed. The dining room can be set up in cabaret style, with table decorations and candlelight. A special dinner is served, followed by the entertainment. Residents, staff and volunteers are invited to perform individual or group items: musical, comical, theatrical or questionable in nature.

Ideas include short skits, resident serenades, ballet performed by male staff, international dancing, recitations, variations on the themes of popular songs, and musical recitals. It is not usually necessary to seek outside entertainment — rely on your own wealth of talented people.

These events require much forward planning and preparation and a planning committee is advisable to organise the various aspects of the evening. It is usually well worth the effort.

At the larger Queen Elizabeth Geriatric Centre, the QE Theatre Group has been formed. This group draws on all sections of the staff and interested residents and performs one or two productions each year. Each section is responsible for at least one act for the concert which is held on three consecutive days so that as many residents as possible can attend. Quite an impressive effort! And very popular.

Sports tournaments

Every two years a major sporting event occurs in the larger community — the Olympics or the Commonwealth Games and a sporting tournament can be arranged to coincide with these occasions. This means a huge round robin of activities all morning, culminating in a wheelchair sprint and medal presentations in the afternoon.

Staff: All other work is cancelled for the day. All staff dress in sporting gear and help run the various events. Local high school children also help run some sections. The games open at 10.30am and continue until noon. The lunch break is followed by the big race, medal presentations and afternoon tea.

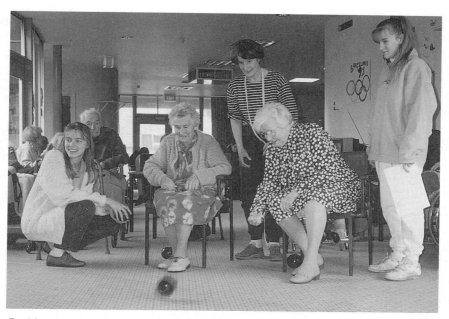

Residents join a huge round robin of sports for the Olympics. Students and the physiotherapist help this team win the bowls section.

Sporting events:

- javelin: rolls of newspaper — distances marked on floor
- basketball: throwing ball into laundry skip frame
- fishing: pick-up stick — 5 differently shaped objects
- target shooting: beanbags or darts
- wrestling: arm wrestles
- weight lifting: various objects of increasing weight
- golf: a mini-golf circuit in garden — objects in garden are aimed for as if they were holes
- soccer: kicking goals into a walking frame
- hockey: upturned walking sticks — hitting goals into walking frame
- wheelchair race: a large die is thrown by participants to move that number of spaces along a course marked out with masking tape. The winner must throw the exact number to win (see 'Cup Day' p. 100)
- swimming could occur on an earlier day at the local pool if some residents attend for aquacise. The physiotherapist could design events for the occasion.

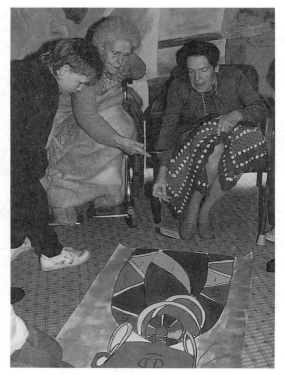

A primary school student helps with the coin tossing.

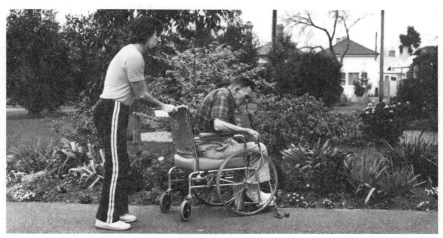

The Executive Director follows instructions as he pushes a golfer around the mini-golf circuit for the Olympic final play-off.

Medal presentation: Gold, silver and bronze chocolate coins (medals) are presented to the decathlon (overall winners) and highest scorers in each event.

Cooking up a cruise

Try turning the entire centre into a cruise ship for a few days and take everyone on a holiday. While some residents are capable of participating in activities outside the centre, others are not. Through this unique idea, you can cater for everyone by, as it were, 'bringing the outside in'. The basic concept is that the premises and daily routine adhere as closely as possible to the appearance and activities associated with an international voyage.

Many hours of planning and cooperation are required from staff, volunteers and residents alike. The cruise will be better managed if certain tasks and responsibilities are delegated to others. Initially, all supporters meet together, then they form sub-committees which establish their own meeting times.

At the initial meetings, the concept of 'brainstorming' ideas is most relevant. Provide the group with a flexible agenda, which covers such areas as:

- cruise destination
- length of holiday or cruise
- appropriate dates
- how best to enjoy ourselves

It is important to keep a record of all the ideas that arise from the brainstorming session. It is surprising the number of wonderful suggestions which can result from collective thinking.

Suggested sub-committees

General promotion: The event will cost money. A raffle can help to fund the events and the local community should also be invited to sponsor the cruise. This can be done through the local media. Press releases to local papers, community announcements on radio and television, and direct approaches to local businesses can all be fruitful.

Ship decorating: There is endless scope for ideas and activities:

- Contact local travel agencies or airline companies for posters, flight display boards, etc.
- Local primary and secondary schools can cooperate by painting murals or making props. This could be done as part of a school assignment, providing plenty of advance notice is given.
- Residents can become significantly involved in many ways — making

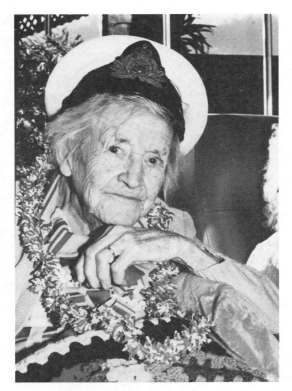

*It's 'Welcome Aboard' to everyone as the
centre gears up for a three-day cruise to Fiji.*

floral leis, designing the ship logo, painting scenes and murals, making collages and prizes for the various on-ship competitions.

Entertainment: The entertainment should complement the theme of the cruise. For instance, a holiday in the tantalising tropics has possibilities for a hula dance and island singing performances; a cruise to the Greek isles could include Greek music and dancing. The need for on-ship entertainment will also provide plenty of options for conventional entertainment. Local personalities, school groups, talented volunteers, residents, staff and community groups are all terrific resources for providing entertainment (see Chapter 9).

Cruise Activities Program: Naturally, all important ships have an official launch. Contact the local mayor or celebrity to crack the champagne bottle over the 'bows'. Streamers, music, a few nibbles and a great sense of fun are the ingredients for success. The captain's cocktail party surely can't be overlooked, and a duty-free shop is a must. (Advertise

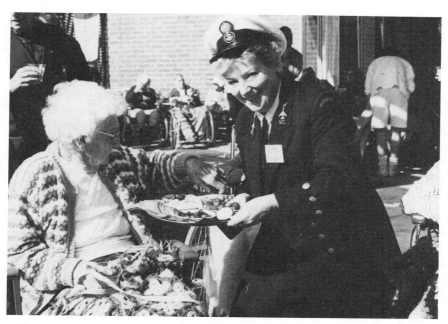

The occasion calls for exotic food, which the crew (staff) help to distribute.

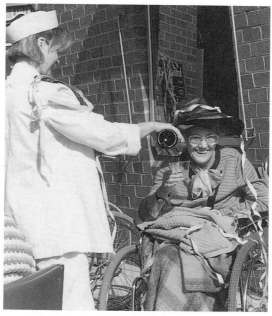

Champagne to toast the ship.

among staff and friends for unwanted bric-a-brac and miscellaneous articles.) Other ideas include a casino night, a ball, a 1960s dance, shipboard games, singalongs, fitness class, life jacket drill, videos and slides.

In order for residents to survive these activities, the daily routine is altered to encourage active participation in the night life. Everyone gets up late, to be ready just in time for the lunchtime activities, which will continue from there into the evening. (Do make sure staff get a few half-hour breaks throughout the day.)

Catering: A travel agent may be able to obtain a ship's menu to guide the selection of dishes. Books from the library and catering colleges will provide handy hints. Residents can take part in baking all the dishes, which may need to be frozen before the big event. A large menu should be displayed listing all the culinary delights over the period of the cruise.

Costumes: Encourage staff to dress up as authentically as possible in shipboard uniform. Hired costumes look effective, but are costly. 'Sailors' look fine in striped T-shirts and long trousers. Residents should be encouraged to wear outfits appropriate to each occasion. Activities could include screen-printing the crew's T-shirt logos. Try making sailor caps with vylene and calico.

Journal: Recording the big event is an integral part of the cruise. Encourage residents to take photographs or write about the voyage. Access to a video camera is a great bonus. Residents, staff and relatives will enjoy repeats of the video with much animation and laughter.

Guest performers

Guest performers — speakers/artists/musicians/creative therapists — can be invited to contribute to the many events described above, or they can constitute the special event themselves. A party afternoon tea can contribute significantly to the atmosphere, and friends and relatives can be invited to attend as well. Special guests can be invited to work with a small group or perform to a large group. Such performers may come just once, or prefer to return regularly to run a variety of events.

Venue: Lounge for large group performances or activities room for group work.

Resources: Refer to Chapter 9 for help in finding guest performers.

Staff: All staff should keep their ears to the ground for local talent.

Preparation activities: Ring around, advertise your need to other staff and involve the residents in the search. Residents may have relatives or friends who know of likely performers. Letters of invitation and thanks will need to be written; some residents may like to assist here. A special afternoon tea can be prepared by residents to add atmosphere and to show

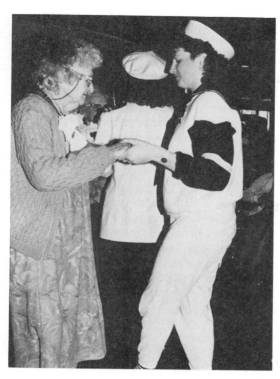

. . . and lots of music and dancing.

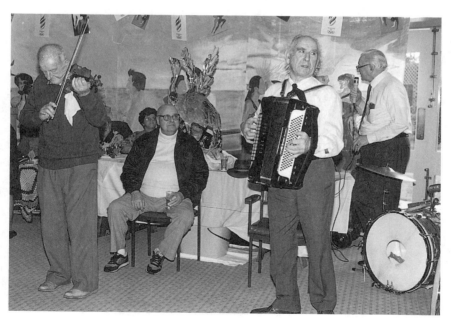

appreciation for the performance. A resident may also like to give a speech of thanks at the end.

Cost: Every attempt should be made to encourage performers to donate their services — offer them food, drink and a very receptive audience, before finally offering money (if you have any available).

Performances might include: Music hall groups; theatrical groups; buskers; dancing — national, ballet, jazz, modern; creative therapy; zoo animals, police dogs and horses, other animals; speakers from various organisations (see Chapter 9 and Appendix A).

Creative therapist: an example

We invited a creative therapist to run a session; he brought a variety of ideas, and was ready to change activities if one was not working. Residents joined in a number of communication games with interest, and generally enjoyed the novel approach. The therapist had brought face paints with him, as they were part of his regular equipment, and asked gingerly if anyone was interested. He was not sure if this age group would consider it appropriate. Surprisingly, some of our most alert residents volunteered to be painted, as long as they could paint some of the staff members' faces

This resident has no qualms about having her face painted.

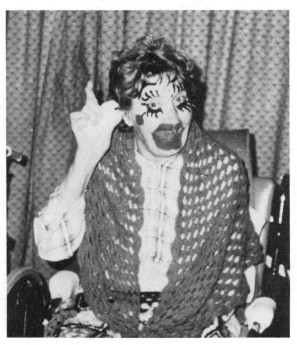

in return. What followed was a great exchange of laughter and joking, and an opportunity for touch and unusual sensory stimulation in a very pleasant, secure atmosphere.

The lesson: never underestimate the interests of residents.

Conclusion

I have heard it said that some special events and parties can be childish and undignified. Some people seem to believe that being a little undignified at times, having fun and socialising is no longer to be considered a normal part of life once one is old. As far as I can tell, most people in the wider community enjoy doing these things; so I can't see why older people should be exempt. Certainly, the residents should determine for themselves the nature and regularity of these events.

The greatest benefits gained from these events include enabling as many people as possible to take part in them, with much resulting laughter. Laughter is a great therapeutic tool and will contribute significantly to the well-being and physical health of residents. In addition, staff morale and therefore the quality of their care for residents will be greatly enhanced if laughter is heard often, from corridors, bathrooms and living areas.

Chapter 6
Outings

Bill had been at South Port for a number of months. He was a delightful but very rigid man, who diligently protected his spot in the lounge room after sitting there for a moment on the first day of his arrival. I would often approach him and invite him to join activities, come on outings, have some fun. But I met constantly with a refusal. I finally said to him: 'Bill, one day, just once, I'm going to get you to say "yes" to me!' Surprisingly, the next time I asked him to join an outing, he laughed and said 'Yes!' It was a trip to the Botanical Gardens.

Bill had lived in Melbourne most of his 85 years, yet had never visited the gardens. He loved them, couldn't get over the size and beauty of the gardens, and particularly enjoyed being pushed up and down the hills by his young attractive volunteer wheelchair pusher.

Since then I have constantly had to persuade Bill to wait his turn to go on outings, and he keeps checking to see if someone has pulled out at the last minute, so that he can take their place. He also joins in far more of the activities at the home. He has discovered that adventure and new experiences are still possible at 85, after a stroke, and living in a nursing home.

Bill, who is now 88, recently visited Lake Mountain, where he saw and touched snow for the first time in his life. He loved it!

The value of outings

It is important to provide opportunities for residents to get out of the confines of the home as often as possible. It gives them the chance to experience the same lifestyle as those who live in the wider community. Outings can simply be a walk down to the local park or milkbar, or major excursions to places of interest or theatrical performances. No one's chances to venture out should be limited, regardless of their age and disabilities.

A wide variety of options needs to be provided to meet the special interests of individual residents. This may mean trips organised for only one or two residents, or the need to hire buses to transport a very large group.

Some people will need encouragement to begin venturing out again. A gentle approach which includes getting to know the special interests of the person, planning a small outing to a relevant venue, and the involvement of a close friend, will help the more reticent person to participate. Very few of the people that I have taken out have refused to go out again. Most of those who decline involvement have yet to try going on an outing. However, some people simply do not like going out, and that's okay. Each person's wishes should be respected.

'At all times staff must be diligent in their supervision of the participants without impeding their independence, enjoyment or dignity'.[1]

Outings can be the most exhausting and most rewarding activities to organise, but they should occur at least fortnightly, preferably weekly, depending on the group size and the effort required to organise each outing. Volunteer and other staff assistance is necessary.

Staff and volunteers

Staff usually include the activity coordinator and/or physiotherapist, assistant, a nurse and volunteers. This will of course vary, depending on the size and nature of the trip. Trips which only require participants to move from the bus to one destination may need only one staff or volunteer to three wheelchair users, whereas a tour or walk will require a 1:1 ratio of

Life continues to be full of adventure. For some, it is their first trip to the snow.

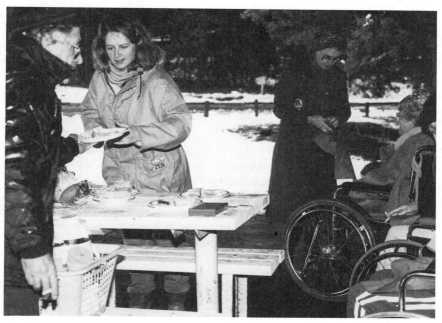

wheelchair pushers and users. Most ambulant residents will need a wheelchair if walking long distances.

It is usually best to restrict transferring and toileting to trained staff. Hence, at least one nursing and/or physiotherapy staff member or assistant is usually required in addition to the activity coordinator, to share these tasks. Volunteers can assist with wheelchair pushing, driving and food distribution.

Equipment

Access to a wheelchair bus is necessary. Your local council or hospital may have one available for use.

Wheelchair buses can also be hired from organisations which cater to the needs of people with various disabilities, such as the Yooralla Society. They usually provide their own drivers and charge for their services. Bookings need to be made well ahead and should be limited to times outside the usual daily schedule of the organisation's own program.

(Mazda Australia, as part of their sponsorship program, donated an 18-seater bus to our nursing home. They also paid for the alterations required for wheelchair transport. We asked them to donate it to the two local councils, who share in the maintenance and storage of the vehicle. It was then available for other groups to book on an occasional basis, too.)

Licence

Most buses require a driver with a heavy endorsement to her or his licence and a passenger certificate. Anyone with such a licence can teach others or, if no such person is available, the first driver can attend a truck driving school and then teach others. It's best to have a number of volunteer bus drivers available, too.

Size

Many buses will carry five wheelchair and five seated passengers. The number of residents who go on an outing varies according to the venue and the number of wheelchair pushers available. You can sometimes take five residents and five wheelchair pushers, for example, or ten residents and use other transport to carry the necessary volunteers.

Cars are usually adequate for very small group outings. Most wheelchair users find the front passenger seat the easiest to get into, as the door opens more widely and there is more leg room.

Other requirements

- The venue needs to be checked beforehand for wheelchair access throughout the facility, particularly toilets.

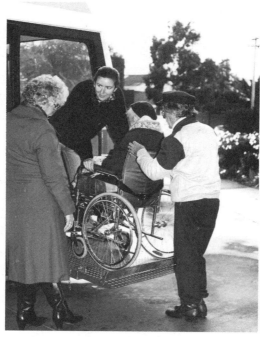

*A nurse, relative and volunteer help to load
the bus for an outing.*

- Many facilities require prior warning of arrival so they can make arrangements for access and seating if needed. They will often make special arrangements for the parking of vehicle/s.
- Lists of names must be distributed to the nurses, kitchen and administration a couple of days ahead, to give plenty of warning. In some cases, outing forms will need to be submitted to the administrative department for approval a few days ahead.
- If necessary, arrangements must be made with the Director of Nursing for a nurse to be available to attend the trip. Sometimes, domestic or administrative staff are invited to join outings, if their work permits.
- Lunch or refreshments need to be arranged. This may mean taking sandwiches and thermos flasks or buying lunch at the venue.
- Money for residents to spend must be arranged from their trusts, or some petty cash from fundraising may be all that is needed, to buy ice-creams, for example.
- An emergency bag with suntan lotion, insect repellent, a urinal bottle, change of underwear and towel is a good idea.

Some extra tips.[1]

- Ensure the residents are dressed appropriately and satisfactorily groomed.
- Women in wheelchairs must have a sufficiently long skirt or knee rug to ensure modesty.
- Wheelchairs must be selected the day before the event so that they are clean, have air in the tyres, and do not need other maintenance.
- If incontinence is a potential concern, check to see if any diuretics can be omitted the previous night or that morning. Ensure that protective garments are worn, and find out the customary timing and frequency of toileting and make every effort to see that it is maintained.
- Only staff trained in transfer and lifting skills should assist in transferring people from car/bus to chair or toilet.

Plan ahead: Each trip will have its own special requirements depending on the venue, the size of the group, the individual residents who participate, and the nature of the activities once there. Each will require careful planning and forethought to ensure that everything goes smoothly.

Be prepared: Make a checklist of requirements beforehand and go through it before leaving. Be prepared to be flexible. Consider alternative venues if the weather is bad; for example, forget the gardens and go to the nearest shopping complex which has a pleasant café and good opportunities for window shopping.

Ideas

Parks and gardens, pubs, galleries, musicals, films, tours. Visit the art centre, a local bay or river mouth by boat, new city building complexes, shopping centres, exhibitions, parades, historic monuments, museums, the market, the zoo. Go fishing, or tour the resident's own old stamping ground. Day trips could include a visit to the mountains or hills nearby, national parks and scenic areas. Many country towns have tourist attractions, such as reconstructed colonial townships, a castle, miniature cities, farming, food production or animal display centres. Special interest groups may like to visit a venue relevant to their topic of interest. Others may wish to attend local community groups, such as neighbourhood groups, day centres, community art or education programs, bowling and senior citizen clubs.

All these venues are very popular. A good cup of coffee, ice-cream or lunch is usually all that is needed to add that finishing touch to the pleasure of these trips.

Country centres

A centre which is based in a country area may have a slightly different range of venues available to it. The Queen Elizabeth Centre, Ballarat

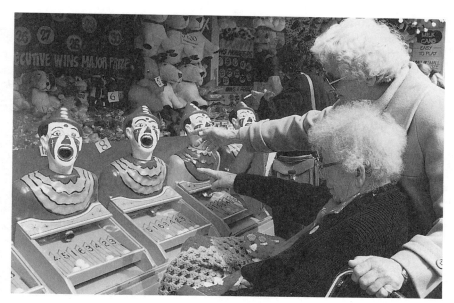

The Royal Show is always a popular outing.

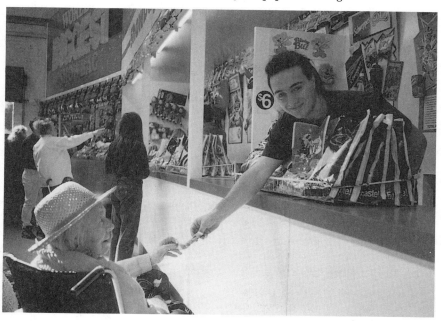

(QEC,B) in country Victoria includes outings to local events such as the country show, local races, begonia festival, local gardens and picnic spots, fishing trips, cricket and football matches, counter lunches at country hotels, church or community group meetings and theatre productions.

Festivals

Many country towns have a local festival which can become the focus for outings and activities. QEC,B involvement in the Ballarat Begonia Festival and their local show illustrate the scope of activities which can become available.

The begonia festival is a big event for residents at QEC,B and involves these activities:

- Day trips to gardens to view begonias (1 staff to 1 resident).
- Painting banners for street decorations organised by a community artist.
- QEC,B enters a float in the procession — residents make paper begonias to decorate it and some participate in the display on the float.
- As many residents as possible (about 200) are taken to the Botanic Gardens to view the procession and enjoy a picnic lunch.
- Small groups attend special activities during festival week, such as concerts, exhibitions and the local prize-winning private gardens.

The local show involves trips lasting 2 hours to view the show activities (1 staff to 1 resident), and residents enter craft in the open, senior citizens and handicapped sections of the show. Participants usually win some prizes in all sections which is good for morale and allows them to compare their work with that of people within the wider community.

Where to get information

Departments of Conservation, Forestry and Lands: Their information centres can provide details of access and facilities at the various national parks and public areas. Look also in the State Government list in your telephone directory for the National Parks and Wildlife Services.

Water Board or an authority such as Board of Works: information can be gained about services and access to a wide range of parkland areas. Look in the State Government section of the telephone directory.

Multi-purpose taxis designed to carry wheelchairs are available from most taxi companies and special discounted rates are available in Victoria, New South Wales, South Australia and the Australian Capital Territory. These discounts can be arranged through the relevant ministry of transport or road traffic authority in each State. In other States, the taxis can be hired through the taxi companies at the normal rate.

State tourist bureaus in each State will direct inquirers to venues accessible to wheelchair users and also offer good information on places of interest available to everyone (see Appendix A).

Disability information services have a comprehensive knowledge of all the recreational venues available in each State (see Chapter 9 and Appendix A for further details).

Conclusion

Outings are fun and most people love the opportunity to get out and have a good look around the local community. Some will resist the idea if they have not been out for a long time, but they can be encouraged. Get to know the individual and find out his or her real interests; plan an outing with these in mind and encourage the person to come and bring along a friend or relative. This gentle approach may be the beginning of a whole new vista of experiences for that person.

Reference

1. Jones M. *Resource Manual, Queen Elizabeth Centre, Ballarat (QEC,B)*. Unpublished manual, 1986.

Further reading

Byrne B. *93 Outings for People who have Trouble Getting Out*. Vantage House, Melbourne 1982. A very useful resource.

Chapter 7
Holidays

We thought disaster had struck when we decided to take Molly to Marysville for a holiday. The winding mountain roads were too much for her tender stomach, despite the precautionary Stemetil supply. She was quite sick and drowsy during the drive and took some time to recover once we reached our destination. She spent most of the next two days sitting on a couch next to her dear friend. They snuggled up asleep on each other's shoulder, sharing a few knee rugs to keep warm, seemingly unaware of the new surroundings and activities happening around them. Molly seemed to enjoy the special meals, yet beyond that . . . she was first to bed and last to rise, and stayed put on her couch during the day.

Most of the other residents had a wonderful time, visiting the falls, playing board games, watching the Marx Brothers, staying up late with the staff, drinking a little too much, joining singalongs — doing all the things which made it obvious they were enjoying themselves. But not Molly. Our dear confused friend seemed even more confused by her new surroundings and chose to shut them out . . . or so it seemed.

We dosed her enough to enable her to travel home free of sickness, but she seemed to sleep all the way. We thought, 'Well, we all make mistakes. We'll know next time.' And certainly we were mistaken. On her return, all Molly could talk about was her wonderful trip to Marysville, and how she hoped so much that her sickness hadn't caused too much trouble.

Molly lived for another six months. She rarely took part in activities as she felt unwell or too tired. Yet every time I spoke to her, even days before she died, she would remind me of her wonderful trip to Marysville and the bus ride over the hills.

The value of holidays

The trip to Marysville is a fairly typical annual holiday during which residents can enjoy the same holiday pleasures as other people in the community. As holidays are a normal activity for most people, they are essential in helping to create a normal home atmosphere at the aged care facility. They provide something very special to look forward to and a way of marking the time of year. A holiday is particularly good for

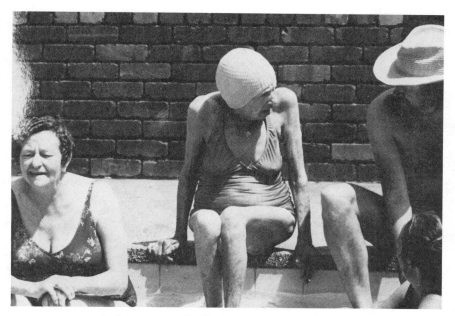

A chance to cool off in the pool at Marysville.

involving relatives and friends in the lives of the residents, as it gives them the opportunity to resume many of their old roles which may have been relinquished to the staff at the home. It also offers a change of environment, new scenery and a source of varied experiences.

Holidays create a more informal atmosphere between staff and residents, helping to break down some of those traditional role models which many residents feel they must attribute to staff. Residents feel able to stay up late, and to talk more freely with the staff and their friends. They assume less of a patient role, a characteristic which even the best nursing home sometimes has difficulty avoiding.

Large annual holiday

Depending on the size of the facility, it is worth taking 15–20 residents, their relatives and friends, volunteers, school children and staff on an annual holiday — a total of about 50 people.

The usual trip will last two nights and three days, with a variety of picnics, outings and activities to fill the days. It is a mammoth task to organise, so plenty of warning and preparation time is needed before the departure date. However, all the hours of work and preparation are worth it for the value which is gained from these holidays.

The options throughout Australia are very broad. Refer to Chapter 9

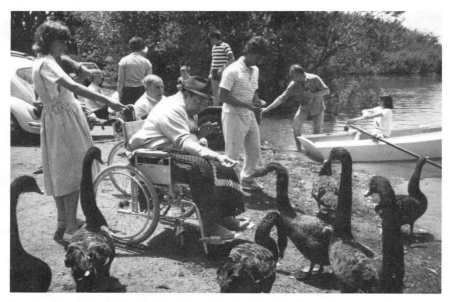

Feeding the barbecue leftovers to the swans at Ballarat Lake.

and Appendix A for ideas on where to go. Holidays could include trips to the seaside, the mountains, river side, farming holidays, historic villages and towns, nearby islands and other tourist attractions. Community-based people unable to go on a holiday alone can also be invited to come along.

Smaller holidays

Such large holidays are annual events, because of their sheer size and organisational demands, but smaller group holidays can be arranged more frequently. Going away in smaller groups also best reflects the style of holiday most people would have experienced in the past.

The venue could be a holiday house anywhere, as long as it is accessible to wheelchairs throughout. A small group of residents, friends and staff can arrange a short holiday at low cost. Everyone can share in meal preparations, while one or two meals could be eaten out at the local pub or restaurant. As these holidays are cheap to organise, they are more accessible to residents with fewer financial resources.

Your centre may be lucky enough to have a friend with a house at the beach or in the mountains which can be used for a number of small trips away. It is worth checking out the availability of free houses before deciding to rent one. These holidays require similar organisational procedures to larger holidays, but the smaller size significantly reduces the effort involved.

Holiday assessment team

In preparation for a holiday, it is worth establishing a holiday assessment team comprising a small group of residents who can regularly visit various holiday resorts to assess their suitability for residents' needs. The group can look at the recreation facilities, type of accommodation and wheelchair accessibility, as well as gain an overall feel for the atmosphere of the place. The trips can include a pub lunch to rest the weary travellers. These trips provide a good excuse for longer outings, and give residents a keen sense of being involved in the planning of their holiday.

Planning the holiday

Time of year: What activities best suit the time of year? Choose venues which will make the most of the seasonal weather. A cosy lounge area with a fireplace and good indoor recreational facilities are ideal for winter trips, while a swimming pool and a variety of nearby outdoor attractions will be great in summer.

Distance is an important consideration: I have found that most older people feel 1–2½ hours' drive is enough, even with a break. A single destination with a variety of tourist attractions is also much easier to organise and more comfortable than a bus tour over a few days.

A chance for old friends to catch up in the relaxed atmosphere of a holiday away.

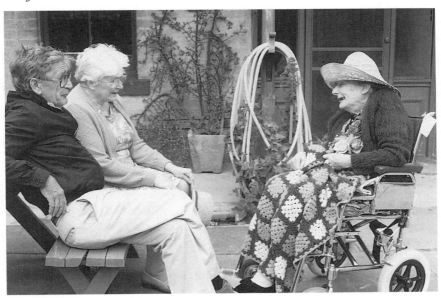

Suitable accommodation: Is the resort fully wheelchair accessible, including the toilets? Are beds easy to transfer people in and out of? Will portable toilet rails be needed? Are the bedrooms off an indoor corridor which would enable a night nurse to offer services to participants? (Some residents will not be able to attend the holiday if a night nurse is not available.)

Recreation facilities: Consider the activities which the resort offers and other equipment which may need to be taken. For example, does the resort provide table games, film projector or video and movies; table tennis and billiards; bar and snack provisions? Is there a variety of recreational areas so that people with different interests can pursue them without inconveniencing others? What nearby tourist attractions will be most likely to interest the group?

Transport: Many bus companies hire out large buses with a hoist for wheelchair users and they usually provide a driver who will participate in all the holiday activities. Alternatively, a number of smaller community buses and cars may be used to reduce costs, particularly for smaller trips.

A flexible itinerary: Contact venues for information on accommodation and outings. Plan alternative activities in case the weather is bad or some activities take longer than expected. In three days, a barbecue picnic on the way there, games and films in the evening, a major outing over lunch on the second day, singing and dancing that night, and a picnic lunch at a place of interest before beginning the journey home on the final day is usually enough to satisfy everyone's desire for an active holiday. (One year it rained continuously, yet we still enjoyed ourselves watching movies, playing games and singing songs. The different location, the familiarity between staff and residents, and the relaxed atmosphere were enough to make the holiday a success.)

Most residents find three days enough and look forward to the familiarity of home, regardless of the enjoyment they may have had while away. Some particularly active residents, however, may prefer a longer holiday and this is best organised with a smaller group of friends and staff. Staff resources will be stretched to the limit over a three-day holiday, so longer trips do become expensive and more difficult to arrange.

Staff/resident ratio: We invite staff from all departments, but everyone assumes responsibility for the complete care of those residents assigned to them. Include a night nurse. The centre meets the cost of staff who attend the holiday. A ratio of one staff to 2–3 residents is usually adequate, although this will vary with the level of dependency of the participants. Volunteers and relatives will be needed to bring this ratio up to 1:1 for wheelchair pushing on excursions.

Cost to residents: Where possible, the home can subsidise the costs for some residents so that they are not excluded through financial constraints. A fundraising drive may be necessary.

Invitations: Relatives and volunteers are invited as guests on the holiday and will need to pay similar rates to the residents. They may wish to help with wheelchair pushing, some personal care for close relatives, and picnic distribution. However, all should find the time away a chance for holidaying and fun, even if not particularly restful. School students who regularly attend the centre may also like to go on the holiday. Their school may be willing to help meet their costs.

Authority forms: Distribute medical and personal authority forms. Ensure that each resident's doctor and, where necessary, their family are aware of the person's decision to participate.

Spending money: Arrange for residents to have money available for personal use.

Room allocation: Obtain a floor plan of the facility and allocate rooms ahead of time.

Bus seating: Devise a bus seating plan well ahead, one which considers people's mobility needs and preference for companionship, and where possible stick to it. This will help to keep track of people and increase the ease and efficiency of loading wheelchair users.

Equipment to include:

- Linen — Continence sheets and other protective bed linen, towels, face washers, continence aids, spare underwear, plastic rubbish bags.
- Travel bag with wet cloth, cups, drinks, sweets, travel pills, spill cloths.
- Picnic equipment: barbecue tools, umbrellas, food and drink, insect repellent, suntan lotion.
- First aid box and each resident's essential drugs.
- In-house equipment — knee rugs, bed socks, toilet aids, walking frames/ sticks, wheelchairs, torches, labels for rooms and luggage, games. Take along a good supply of snacks and a variety of beverages for supper and midnight snacks.

What to look for in a resort

One centre that the assessment team visited and subsequently chose for a holiday had several features which made it attractive.

The resort was just two hours' drive away and located opposite a major historical attraction. It had a self-contained lodge with accommodation for about 50 people. It was completely wheelchair accessible, although the toilets did not have rails or aids. All bedrooms led off a central corridor, enabling night supervision. A comfortable recreation area offered billiards, music, games, and a relaxation area. Main meals were eaten in the next building, which was a ballroom, and provided a special treat for residents.

The facility provided an uncooked breakfast in the lodge, cut lunches for the picnics, and a three-course dinner for the evening meal in the ballroom. They offered several menus which varied in price, enabling us to select attractive meals while remaining within our budget.

Activities could include a barbecue lunch on the way there, a visit to the historical village the next day, then lunch in the gardens before leaving for home on the third day.

This demonstrates the basic requirements of a good holiday resort — we had a great time as a result.

Where to get ideas

ACROD is a disability information service which will give you details about accessible venues for trips (see Disability Information Services in Appendix A). ACROD also produces a booklet called *Room 206: Accommodating Travellers with Disabilities*. It sets out the design requirements for hotels and motels which will facilitate their use by people with disabilities, and it is distributed to holiday facilities throughout Australia. It is also available from ACROD. It is designed to encourage many more holiday facilities to cater for the needs of the disabled, and should broaden the range of choices available for holiday venues.

Tourist Bureau travel centres will direct inquirers to venues accessible to wheelchair users and other disabled people. They also offer good information about general places of interest available to everyone. If you know where you want to go, and indicate your specific needs for access and assistance, these centres can make the necessary arrangements to ensure hassle-free travel. Most have listings of the accessibility ratings of accommodation and tourist resorts to help your planning (see Appendix A).

The Railway Package Tour Department can be contacted in each State through the State Rail Authority. It provides information about tour options and will make sure all the special needs of your group are catered for.

The Helping Hand service provides assistance for people travelling by train. Once the destination is known The Helping Hand can be contacted to arrange for someone to be available at the platform to assist in whatever way is necessary. The service is available for day trips and holidays. For example, they will arrange help at stations to purchase tickets, find correct platforms, and book multi-purpose taxis. It is a particularly useful service for the individual wheelchair traveller.

Bus tours: Many bus companies now have some buses with wheelchair facilities — most travel agencies can direct you to them. Some actually specialise in tours for the disabled, adventure weekends and contract tours. Some also offer specialised programs for older people.

See Chapter 9 and Appendix A for further information and resources.

Conclusion

Holidays are wonderful for breaking down barriers between staff and residents and the relaxed atmosphere enhances the development of close friendships between all involved. (It's good to see a resident sitting up long into the night with staff and volunteers, sharing in the discussions and inevitable gossip.) This change in roles can have lasting positive effects on the relationships between these groups when they return home and, for this reason alone, the trips are well worth the effort.

Chapter 8

Music

by Mary Ward

'Music moves its mountains slowly yet it shapes the soul of man as surely as any other force.'[1]

It was St Andrew's day and the piper had arrived to play the bagpipes. She piped in the haggis, then followed it with a selection of tunes requested by the residents. The unusual sound of the bagpipes seemed to have a power all its own. Many sang along with the tunes, some looked on with rapt attention, while others fought back the tears as the cry of the bagpipes brought old memories flooding back. Even I, who had grown up with rock and roll, felt its power. One man quite openly wept tears of joy as the music played.

Moments later the mood changed as Jock, a piano-accordion player took over the floor and led everyone in many lighthearted songs. Laughter echoed about and joy became the dominant feeling in the room.

Music is a very powerful medium which affects our lives in many ways. Music can be the focus of many activities, or simply the mood setter as background music for special events and some group activities.

Creative use of music

(Mary Ward is a music therapist who works in the area of aged care. A few years ago, her mother had a severe stroke which placed her in a nursing home. So that she could join a 'stimulation group' at the home, Mary also became a member of the stimulation group. She played the piano for singalongs and other musical activities. It soon became clear that music was an excellent stimulator and a wonderful aid to communication and socialisation. This realisation made her change direction; she studied for a postgraduate diploma in Music for Therapy and, since that time, has been involved in using music to improve the quality of life of older people. Mary Ward has contributed the material for this chapter to offer a guide to the use of music in a variety of creative ways.)

A music therapist seeks to bring about therapeutic change in disabled people through the planned and controlled use of music. However, many people simply provide music for pleasure within aged care facilities and need new ideas for musical activity groups. The ideas presented here will help to vary the music program for these people. The aim is to show how music can become a greater part of the activity program, rather than to discuss its application as a therapeutic tool.

Musical preferences

Music is a very associative medium and a familiar tune often brings back memories. Many elderly people, when they were young, carried out much of their communication and socialisation while singing round the piano. So music remembered from their youth can often revive old memories, stimulating the mind and bringing back communication and social skills which may have fallen into disuse.

It is important, therefore, to consider the musical tastes of the group and to be aware of the particular songs and music from their eras (see Appendix F for well-known songs from different eras). Those born in the early 1900s will probably be familiar with the songs of the twenties because of their parents' choice of music; they will know the 1930s' tunes because of their own preferences, and possibly those of the 1940s through the favourites of their children. This gives a wide range of music and song to use with older people.

Most residents will have varying preferences in the style of music. Some will prefer the classics, others jazz and blues, and still others will prefer middle of the road, easy listening music. Most residents choose to have the latter playing in communal areas. It is therefore important to offer participants the chance to form their own musical appreciation groups. It is also worth noting that few older people like loud, hard rock; it can be very aggravating, particularly for those with a hearing loss. It simply becomes a thumping beat which drowns out other sounds. Residents must always have control over the selection of music being played for them.

The value of musical activities

The value and power of music is infinite. Most people are aware of the great range of effects music can have on them. It can make them happy or sad, cause them to laugh or cry, dance or relax; it can change moods. Music can motivate, aggravate, stimulate the mind, cause spontaneous uncontrollable reflexes and help improve coordination. It can be beneficial to respiratory and digestive functions and also reduce anxiety. Some perceptual and emotional musical experiences can lead to changes in blood pressure, pulse rate, respiration and autonomic functions. These physical

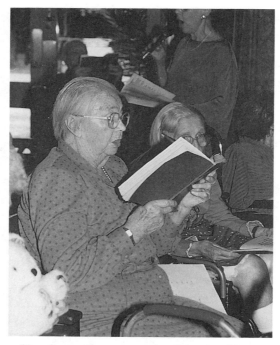

*Singalongs draw out and affirm the skills of
many residents.*

functions become synchronised with the flow of the music, and music is
now being recognised as a powerful tool for fostering good health.

Communication

A major benefit of the use of music can occur in the area of communication. Some people with communication disorders begin to communicate
again through musical activities. Ethel, who had not spoken with anyone
in recent years, chose to join the music group. She gradually began to
communicate with the music therapist and then other members of the
group through talking and singing. The music provoked something within
Ethel which freed her to begin communicating with others again.

Self-esteem

Music activities can also provide many opportunities for improving self-
esteem. Many people who have lost their speech due to a stroke or brain
damage are still able to sing familiar songs, and this can work wonders for
their self-confidence.

Those who find it difficult to join in more active groups can choose
their own level of involvement in a music session. There is room for a

person just to be part of the group, listening and enjoying the atmosphere, without feeling the need to perform. The emphasis is on enjoyment.

Emotional relief

Musical activity can offer a chance for people to release their frustrations. Percussion instruments can provide a socially acceptable way of 'bashing away' pent-up emotions. Players are able to 'say' just what they think, in a non-verbal way, on a percussion instrument, without actually addressing anyone or hurting their feelings.

Creativity

We are all creative beings and music is an excellent avenue through which to explore our creativity in improvisation, composition, art and dance. Such exploration into the creative self will contribute to self-esteem, expression of feelings, and the ability to communicate creatively with others.

Physical exercise

Many older people are quite averse to physical exercise and music is valuable for the way it can motivate them to participate. If the emphasis is placed on the musical activity rather than the exercise, many will take part enthusiastically and have been known to comment later: 'That *was* good exercise, wasn't it!' (see also Chapter 4 for movement to music ideas.)

Approaching the person with dementia

Music is an excellent medium to use to communicate with confused people. However, it should be used in a very gentle, sensitive manner. Confused people respond well to musical activity if they are accepted as they are with a loving, caring attitude. They can be fully absorbed in a music group for over an hour (see also Chapter 14).

Flo was a resident who seemed happy in her dementia. In working with her, the overall aim was to improve her communication skills by singing songs from her past. Part of this involved encouraging her to recall events connected with the songs and, from there, to draw her gradually into the present. Flo responded well, she enjoyed herself, and her communication, memory and respiration all improved. Yet she indicated that she was aware of the aim to reorient her to the real world. She made it known that she was happy in her fantasy world and did not wish to leave it.

While some people with dementia prefer to live in their fantasy world, it is important to offer activities like music which give them a chance to leave it behind and return to reality, if they so choose. Music also provides some measure of quality of life for the participants, regardless of the choice they make.

Musical activities

Most of the musical activities listed below are appropriate for both alert people and those with memory loss. They have been specifically designed for non-ambulant people, but they are all suitable for ambulatory people as well. Any number can participate in each activity.

There is a need to be flexible with the programs. People vary from day to day, and what suits one group of people may not necessarily be relevant to another group. The leader must tune into the feelings of the group and be prepared to change the planned activity as needed.

Seating arrangements

Wherever possible, have the people in the group sitting in a circle. In this way, everyone can maintain eye contact and the leader can be aware of each individual's reactions.

Singalongs

Never underestimate the value of a singalong. A person's most intimate means of self-expression is the voice, and singing is the original form of musical self-expression. The voice could be said to be a built-in musical instrument. Usually older people enjoy singing, especially songs which are familiar to them. Even though they may say they can't sing or read the words, you will usually find they forget their supposed limitations and join in. Some enjoy just being in a singing group, even if they don't sing.

Conversation may be stimulated through past association with familiar songs. After singing a song, the leader can gently guide people into chatting about memories the song may have evoked, or just talking about the ideas stimulated by the songs.

Words: The Ulverscroft large print song books[2] are very useful. They are easy to hold and most people can read the large print. Many older people find single song sheets difficult to hold. The song books encourage people to find the numbers and the songs. Each person can be invited to choose a song for the group to sing. If residents take turns round the circle, they begin to anticipate their turn and have a song ready. Participants who may be less alert will sometimes develop these skills of selection over time, demonstrating improvement in their awareness of their surroundings.

Themes: Singalongs are often most enjoyed if based on a theme, for example, Australiana. The scene could be set with gum-tree tips decorating the room, swaggie hats and, if possible, billy tea and damper. Reminisce about the 'good old days', drawing on the older person's wealth of experience and information. This contributes significantly to their sense of

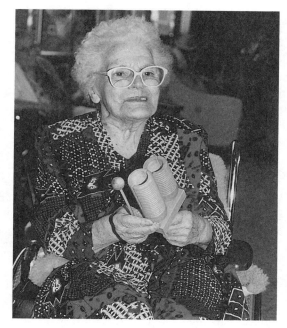

A group meets regularly to share and create music.

worth and increases self-esteem (see Chapter 5 for calendar themes and Appendix F for song titles suited to various themes).

Rounds: Singing in rounds can be fun. Choose songs such as 'Kookaburra sits in the old gurn tree', 'Frère Jacques', 'Row, row, row your boat', and 'Oh, how lovely is the evening'.

Action songs can provide exercise and lots of fun as well (see Appendix F for ideas).

Music appreciation

Listening to music is pleasurable in itself. In the communal environment it is often difficult to listen to music without interruption, and people with differing tastes need chances to listen to their preferred music (see Chapter 4 for music appreciation group suggestions).

Music for entertainment

Musical entertainment of any kind is always very popular. Guest performers or talented staff, residents and volunteers may like to present a concert or musical recital. The performance can be an event in itself or part of a larger special event (see Chapter 5 for entertainment ideas for special events and Chapter 9 for a guide to finding entertainers).

Background music

Music can be a good mood-setter. Pleasant, bright music can enhance the atmosphere of some group activities — it may set the scene for an expressive art group, for instance. However, it should be at a comfortable volume which does not interfere with conversation. Background music should be avoided with people with significant hearing loss or confusion. Group members themselves should decide if and what they will listen to while participating in an activity.

Musical passing games

Listed below are popular games which have been adapted by adding music. In each case, the group sits in a circle, singing and passing round an object while bright, familiar music is played. When the music stops, the player holding the object either throws it, unwraps it or drops out.

It is possible to develop or adapt many other games to make them more suitable for a particular group. The games should be matched to the functional level of the group members to ensure that participants succeed at the tasks.

While residents are involved in the activities, a number of processes occur which:

- improve physiological functions
- stimulate memory
- increase focus of attention and concentration
- stimulate thought processes, communication and social interaction
- boost self-esteem and self-confidence
- enhance reality orientation
- provide opportunity for exercise

All this is in addition to the fun and pleasure gained from participating in the activities.

Basic equipment

Each activity needs the following basic equipment:

- a hand-held cassette player, worked by the group leader (or, if possible, a musician to play the music)
- bright music, familiar to the group
- two sets of differently coloured streamers, if the game is to be played in teams

Musical noughts and crosses (tic tac toe)

Equipment:

- large piece of non-slip fabric (curtain lining is ideal), divided into 9 squares with a marking pen
- 4 green beanbags, each marked with an X
- 5 orange beanbags, each marked with an O
- orange and green ribbons for each member of the group
- tape of stimulating songs familiar to the group

Procedure:

- Each alternate person in the circle displays a green or orange ribbon to indicate their team.
- Place the grid on the floor in the centre of the circle.
- The leader plays the music tape while the group members sing and pass 2 beanbags (one green, one orange) round the circle. When the music stops, the participants holding the beanbags throw them onto any 1 of the 9 spaces on the grid.
- Repeat this process until there is a complete row of 3 Os or Xs.

If a person from one team ends up with the opposition's bag when the music stops, she can try to throw the bag where it will avoid making a line for the other team. (Or she may prefer to help them!) Keep a score of the number of games won.

Note: Some people function better if they play in pairs rather than teams. Some confused people grasp only the concept of throwing the bag onto a square. Invariably, the more aware people win the game, but they are usually ready to help each other. If the game is not made too competitive the emphasis will be on everyone participating and having fun.

Hangman

Equipment:

- white board and pen or blackboard and chalk
- picture of a hangman (if you don't know what the hangman looks like ask someone else!)
- a beanbag
- tape of stimulating music, familiar to the group

Procedure:

- Ask one of the participants to give you a word in private, preferably a noun.
- Draw a line of dashes on the board, one for each letter. e.g. _ _ _ _ _ _

- Pass the beanbag to the music. When the music stops the participant holding the beanbag calls out a letter. If that letter occurs in the word it is written above the appropriate dash. For each letter called out which does not occur in the word, the leader draws a part of the hangman picture. The incorrect letters are recorded so participants can see which letters have already been tried. The person who completes the word before the hanged man is completed chooses the next word.

The game can be played using themes such as first names, book titles, etc.

Pass the ball

This game can be played in teams or individually.

Equipment:

- 2 large foam balls
- 2 medium foam balls
- 2 small foam balls
- 1 or 2 buckets
- tape of stimulating songs familiar to the group
- 2 sets of ribbons of different colours to mark teams

Procedure:

- Participants sit in a circle with the buckets in the centre. (If playing in teams, distribute the 2 colours to each alternate person.)
- Pass the 2 large balls around as participants sing to the music. When it stops, those holding the balls throw them into the buckets. The smaller balls are used as the players become more proficient. A score can be kept to encourage competition, although to many the challenge of getting the ball in the bucket is enough.

Variation: The ball is passed round; the person left holding the ball when the music stops is out.

Velcro Darts

Equipment: Velcro Darts set; or a felt dartboard and 2 foam balls with strips of velcro round them.

Procedure:

- The dartboard can be held or transported on a wheelchair.
- The 2 velcro balls (darts) are passed round together to the music. When the music stops the participant holding the 2 balls throws them. Scores are kept.

Hookey, skittles and bowls can also be played in this manner.

Pass the parcel

Equipment:

- A parcel made with as many wrappings as people in the group. Between each layer include an instruction either to sing a song, or tell a story or joke. Put a prize in the centre. Alternatively, include messages for the person with the most beautiful eyes, the most handsome gentleman, etc.
- Tape of stimulating songs, familiar to the group.

Procedure:

- the group sings to the music while the parcel is passed round
- when the music stops, the participant holding the parcel unwraps one layer and follows the instructions
- this continues until someone wins the prize

Spin the bottle

Equipment:

- a bottle
- a bucket containing messages with instructions to tell a story or joke, mime an action, sing a song, etc.
- tape of stimulating songs familiar to the group

Procedure:

- pass the bottle round while everyone sings to the music
- when the music stops, the person who has the bottle spins it
- whoever the bottle points to takes a message and follows its instructions

The group can vote for the most original act — with a full bottle as the prize! Alternatively, some members may like to play the authentic version to music!

Concentration

Equipment:

- a magnetic board
- 12 magnets
- tape of stimulating songs familiar to the group
- a beanbag
- a large drawing of a song title, familiar to the group, e.g. 'Roll out the barrel'
- 12 cards marked 1–12 which will, together, cover the song title drawing

On the reverse side of the cards, in large print, write well known song titles. Make two cards for each song title e.g. cards 1 and 9 might have 'Swannee' on the back, while cards 2 and 4 might have 'Clementine' on them.

Procedure:

- Set up the puzzle before the group arrives. The cards are placed over the picture with the numbers showing, held in place with the magnets.
- The beanbag is passed round while the group sings to the music.
- When the music stops, the person holding the beanbag calls out two numbers between 1 and 12. The two numbers are turned over; if they are a pair, the player keeps the cards, scoring one point for each card. That person is then entitled to another turn. (This of course leaves spaces so that part of the song title can be seen.)
- This process is repeated until someone guesses the song title. The correct guesser scores 5 points. The highest scorer wins.

Musico (musical bingo)

A particularly popular game.

Equipment:

- Large bright cards, 30 × 30 cm, divided into 9 squares. One card for each participant (see diagram).

Swannee	Melbourne Town	Rose of Tralee
Waltzing Matilda	Tipperary	Tea for Two
Clementine	Irish Eyes	K-K-Katie

Each square has a well known song title marked on it in large print. On each card, one or two song titles will vary from those on the other cards, so that each card is different.

- Small cards to cover the squares, 9 per person. Large buttons can also be used.
- Smaller cards, each bearing one of the song titles, for the musician's use.
- Musical instrument.
- Prizes.

Procedure:

- Each person is given a song card and 9 cover cards (as for bingo).
- Discuss the prize — it could be 'a world trip', 'a sheep station', a 'Rolls Royce' or a lucky dip.
- The musician's cards are shuffled and placed face down. The first card is turned over and the musician plays the first line of the tune on the card. The group guesses the title, sings the song and covers the title on their card if it matches. The person who covers all their songs first calls out 'Musico' and wins the game.

Note: Many people with confusion can play this game successfully. They may need reinforcement from a helper who can ask if they have 'Clementine' on their card when they miss a song. However, they should be encouraged to cover the song title themselves. Neighbours will often notice missed songs and point them out. This is more likely to occur if a fun, non-competitive atmosphere is fostered. Some who have difficulty at first can eventually learn to play the game successfully.

Detectives

Equipment:

- small articles suitable for hiding
- music familiar to the group

Procedure:

- The group sits in a circle; one of the members leaves the room or is blindfolded. While he is away, the group decides where to hide the 'stolen' object, allowing it to show just a little.
- When the 'detective' returns, the group sings a familiar song; the closer the detective gets to the object, the louder the group sings, the further away, the softer they sing. The person who hid the stolen object becomes the next detective.

Percussion

Percussion instruments can be used in many ways. As mentioned earlier, they can provide a socially acceptable way of expressing anger and frustration. Percussion instruments include various types of drums, sticks,

bells, triangles, maracas, tambourines, castanets, claves, cymbals, blocks
and guiros. If you have insufficient money to buy many instruments, there
are several books available (see end of chapter) which give simple instructions for making such things as claves (from two pieces of dowel), coconut
shells, a wobble board, maracas (from plastic bottles and rice), and a
drum (from a cake tin and heavy plastic).

How to play percussion instruments

Provide an assortment of percussion instruments for the group. Introduce
each one and demonstrate how it is played. Allow group members to
practise playing their instrument correctly, then suggest they try to be
creative and find out how many different ways the instrument can be
played, to discover as many different sounds as possible. For example,
striking the instrument's handle or the side of a drum will make a different
sound. Encourage improvisation. Many people develop a preference for
one type of instrument and may wish to become proficient with it.

Rhythm band: There are many ways of using a rhythm band playing
percussion instruments. It can be as simple as playing along with a musician, tape or record. Alternatively, the group can be divided into sections, with each member in a section playing a similar instrument. Each
section is given a rhythm and asked to work together to accomplish it.
When each group is confident they can play their rhythm, they can all be
put together with music. The performance should be recorded so that
everyone can listen to the overall effect.

Jug band is made up of homemade instruments such as bottles, a wash-
board, pots and pans, and other kitchenware. A makeshift upright bass
can be made from a broomstick placed in the centre of an upside-down
washbasin with a nylon string running from the top of the broomstick to
the edge of the wash basin. Fill bottles with water to different levels to
create a variety of pitches. The bottles can be tapped or blown across the
top to make sounds. Again, record the end result so that everyone can
hear how it sounds. One of the members of the band should fill the
important role of conductor.

Percussion sound effects: The group could write a script for radio
which requires special sound effects for the story. Discuss the theme of the
story. One that is popular is 'The Saga of the Early Morning Sounds
in a Nursing Home'. This gives residents the chance to dispel a certain
amount of frustration about the sounds they hear; it can be channelled
into a very humorous activity. Sounds can be replicated by using the usual
percussion instruments plus pots and pans or whatever else makes the
right sound.

One person reads the story, while the other members make the sound effects at the appropriate times. Tape the story for others. It can be edited as necessary.

Body percussion: Bodies can be used as percussion instruments. Try different sequences of clapping, slapping, clicking and stamping in addition to the other percussion instruments. This can add depth and clearer rhythm to the overall effect of the percussion band.

• experiment with different rhythms, or by changing the order of them
• add variety by chanting a phrase
• beat out rhythms to recorded music; e.g. 'Hooked on classics' provides a good accompaniment for this activity
• each group member could take turns to lead the rest of the group in a body percussion action

Voice percussion: The voice can also be used as a percussion instrument; various voice sounds can be added to the rhythms and instruments to give greater variety, or the voice can also be used alone. An example:

OLD-TIME FAIRGROUND STEAM ENGINE

Group	*Sound*
1. The engine	Um-Pom-Pom (repeatedly)
2. The steam blowing	Um-Sssh-Sssh (repeatedly)
3. The valve	Um-tiddley-AR (repeatedly in falsetto voice)
4. The music	Hold nose while singing la-la to any old tune, e.g. 'The More we are Together'.

Note: Such use of percussion instruments can contribute significantly to improved socialisation, through group interaction and cooperation. It can be a very satisfying and enjoyable experience, providing a positive chance for those with communication difficulties to participate more fully.

Creative movement

Percussion instruments can be used with creative movement and dance. Participants are encouraged to use expressive movements to match the feel of the music or to express an emotion. The movements can be confined to the upper limbs where necessary.

For example: 'Everyone reach up to pick some fruit. Then lower your hand in a way which expresses disappointment or pleasure.' The musical instruments can be used to complement the movements.

This type of creative expression is probably best led by an experienced music therapist or artist. Such a person could be invited to establish a group which could then be taken over by other staff after training. Alternatively, interested staff may like to attend a course to develop skills in the area (see Chapter 9 and Appendix A for resources).

Musical quizzes

(These quiz ideas have been devised by Betty Stinson, an occupational therapist who has specialised in the field of aged care and dementia.)

- follow the themes of the year and ask the group to think of appropriate songs, e.g. Australiana, folklore Irish songs, love songs for St Valentine's day (see Chapter 5)
- ask the group to think of songs which mention colours, animals, flowers, birds, cities of the world, or first names
- ask the group to think of and sing songs from the first and second world wars
- the leader sings the first line of a song, which the group is required to finish

When the group has selected a song, everyone sings it together. Use all these quizzes to encourage reminiscing. Discuss and share the memories they trigger. (Refer to the list of song title categories and the age-related and popular song title lists in Appendix F.)

Why music?

Music can[3]:

- reach any person, bedridden or ambulatory, for it does not always require active participation
- provide a method of communicating with even the most depressed person
- motivate people to take part in physical activity, strengthen muscles and improve motor coordination
- enhance social interaction, improving socialisation and communication skills
- renew interest in attending other social functions, including activities in the community
- increase attention span, by focusing thoughts onto specific, reality-oriented activities
- help people to feel better about themselves, improving their self-concept
- show a way to creative expression through a combination of music, drama, physical movement and rhythmic activity
- assist in appropriate expression of feelings which may otherwise remain suppressed
- provide enjoyment, happiness and stimulation to the mind

- provide relaxation, and deepen and expand consciousness, which may improve mental health

If music can do all these things, then it should form a large part of any activity program designed to improve the quality of life of its participants.

References

1. Fleming and Venus, *Understanding Music*. N.Y. Holt, Rinehart & Winston. 1958.
2. *The Ulverscroft Large Print Song Book*. Ulverscroft Large Print Books Ltd, Leicester, UK.
3. Douglass D. *Accent on Rhythm*. La Roux Enterprises, PO Box 745, Salem.

Further reading

Homemade musical instruments:
Southworth M. *Making Musical Sounds*. Australia: Cassell, 1976.
The Musical Instrument Recipe Book. Penguin, 1968.
Sturman P. *Creating Music*. Harlow. UK: Longman, 1982.

Chapter 9
Links with the Local Community

Our local zoo has an educational unit which gives sessions to groups who visit the zoo. It also provides a service for groups who find it difficult to visit the zoo. The educators bring native Australian animals into the aged care centre and show slides of the zoo. The animals are passed round for residents to touch and look at closely.

Everyone who could crammed into the lounge to see the slides and animals. Passing staff members couldn't help but stop, to cuddle the possum or respond to the dares to touch the snake. The wombat and possum brought great pleasure to everyone, and the snake certainly stimulated interest. One resident quite happily demonstrated her courage by holding Monty the python and letting him slither over her arms. It was a memorable occasion.

The service was invited back six months later. A resident, whose recent memory was considered to be very poor, was told of the imminent return of the zoo visitors. Her response was: 'Oh, will the snake be coming again?' It had obviously made quite an impact on her.

Many such experiences can be made available to residents as links are formed with local community resources.

Community involvement

A successful activities program cannot exist in a vacuum. It must encourage all sectors of the surrounding community to become involved. People with a wide range of personalities and abilities then become available to enrich the lives of residents, far beyond anything the staff, with limited time and skills, can provide. The effort and time devoted to collecting resources from the various services listed in this chapter are repaid many times over by the resulting activity opportunities which become available to residents.

Residents also need to be given the opportunity to go out into the local community to be involved in groups or activities of their choice. Such involvement allows them to exercise their interests in the same way as other members of the community. Some may continue to attend the same clubs or neighbourhood groups as in the past, while other residents can

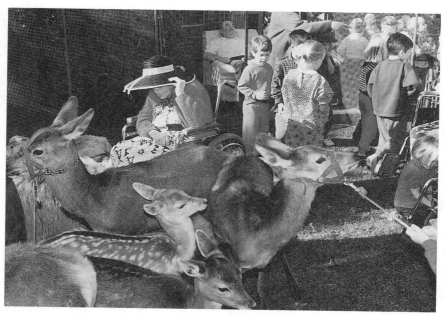

Linking with the community can mean sharing the cost of a visiting zoo with the local kindergarten.

be introduced to new groups, classes and experiences. Such involvement helps to maintain a sense of continuity between the person's former life as a member of the local community and their present circumstances.

A well coordinated volunteer program contributes significantly to this process. A coordinator of volunteers is needed to develop and encourage such volunteer involvement. As government funding is not available for this kind of position, the Management Committee and the Auxiliary may commit themselves to raising such funds, or other trust or employment initiative programs may be drawn upon to supplement the wage required (see Appendix A: Trusts).

In addition to the activity coordinator's position, a coordinator of volunteers requires at least 10–12 hours' working time for a 60-bed home. However, the resultant gain in actual work hours from this expenditure is immeasurable (see Chapter 10).

The activity coordinator and the coordinator of volunteers are able to establish an extensive resource of people and groups who can provide entertainment, drive buses, go on outings and holidays, and run or assist in most activities. They give staff and residents the extra support they need and, perhaps most importantly, they bring the local community into the home.

How to use this chapter

This chapter describes the main agencies to approach to gain information for a resource file, in addition to the local groups who are most likely to be of assistance. The services described will refer the reader to the appendix that lists the interstate addresses of many of them. The reader can also refer to other appropriate chapters to put the combination of resources and activities into practice. No two centres will want the same list of contacts and ideas, and resource lists are quickly out-of-date. Thus, what follows is a general guide to where to go for information, so that each facility can compile a list of resources which is relevant to its clientele and specific to its location.

Establishing a resource file

A card file is a very handy method of recording ideas, outings, guest speakers, entertainers, information services and suppliers. Information can be listed on individual cards in alphabetical order for easy reference and updating. (It is usually easiest to find information listed under the **type** of service, rather than the name of the individual service provider, as names can be forgotten.)

A notice board displaying community resource information for residents, relatives and staff is also a useful way of encouraging residents to involve themselves and their relatives in community activities.

Where to look for help and ideas

In establishing a resource file it is worth contacting Local Government Services first, where the recreation officer can direct inquirers to a wide range of resource material (see Local Government below).

The following information includes a guide to making the most of local community resources, service clubs, disability information agencies, training colleges and peer support groups. Through tapping into all these groups, the activity coordinator will not only have access to valuable information, but she will also find ongoing support and encouragement from a much broader team of workers.

Telephone directory

Many of us do not use the telephone directory to our best advantage. Much of the information we require can be found by a phone call to the relevant government body. Find the section of the telephone directory which gives an index to all government services. Ring up relevant agencies and find out what they can offer your centre.

Local sources

Make the most of your local resources.

Advertise: Display posters locally requesting information about amateur theatrical groups, musical performers, magicians and novelty acts. Advertise in the community announcement section of your local newspaper.

Newspapers: Read local and major papers for coming events and entertainment.

Staff: Encourage all staff to become talent scouts, looking out for anyone with a talent suitable for activities at the centre.

Establish links with other local, interstate or overseas centres and exchange information and ideas. This can be enhanced by visits to other local centres, shared in-service days, communal afternoon teas, and newsletter exchanges. An overseas centre may like to exchange slides and cassette tapes to encourage the sharing of ideas.

Local Government

Most Local Government bodies (shires, boroughs, municipalities, local councils) will have a Municipal Recreation Officer/Community Arts Officer/Leisure Services Officer (their titles can vary greatly) who can direct you to resources in a variety of areas. Their links with local and regional community groups are extensive. Many of the regional groups can then direct you to statewide and national bodies as required. Many local councils also publish their own Community Resource Directory each year.

Most major municipal councils can supply a Mobility Map of the metropolitan area which provides information about access and facilities for people with limited mobility. Ring the Community Services department of the local council for details.

The following services can all be contacted through the Municipal Recreation Officer.

Local library: Most libraries have community resources to lend to groups. They will supply large print books, tapes, pictures, reference books and music relevant to activities; they often also have audiovisual equipment which can be borrowed. A phone call will usually enlist the help of the library staff to research and deliver the material.

Neighbourhood groups: The citizens' advice bureau or local community centre may be able to direct you to groups in your area.

Ethnic community groups: There may be an ethnic community officer employed by the council or borough or a migrant resource centre may exist.

Volunteer centres: There are local, regional and Statewide representative associations for volunteers which can be contacted through the recreation officer. These services offer support and advice to volunteers and also match volunteers to service providers who require their assistance (see Appendix A).

Community Centres and Neighbourhood houses

Make contact with your local community centre or house. These centres usually run a whole range of activities and programs to which you may be able to send residents. They usually offer many different crafts, creative writing, relaxation, travel groups, dances, support groups and more. You may be able to link in with the centre to share ideas, resources and volunteers.

Bowling/senior citizens/service clubs

These groups often have a wealth of talented people available to offer voluntary entertainment or special interest talks to the residents. It is worth developing strong links with these groups to gain regular entertainers and volunteers. It may be possible to visit some of your local clubs and speak at their meetings about the areas of involvement open to them. Many residents may wish to participate regularly in the clubs' activities.

Buskers

Try approaching buskers and invite them to attend the home. We have found some great entertainers this way.

Local business

Advertising, donations and community involvement can all occur through local shops and businesses. All should be encouraged to invest in their local area.

Fashion parades

There are usually plenty of clothing agencies keen to sell their clothes to residents by means of a fashion parade. It is best, however, to try to arrange a deal with a local shop, where prices may be cheaper, and where staff and residents can be models in the parade. This creates much more fun and prevents the hard-sell approach.

Local churches

Many churches have community activities which residents can attend and they are also a good source of volunteers. They may be involved in task-oriented activities which some residents may want to contribute to, increasing opportunities for them to give to others.

Charitable agencies

Many charitable and church agencies have community service divisions which provide a large range of residential services for older people. A worthy exchange of resources and ideas can be established with some of the centres run by these groups. The Uniting Church in Australia has an excellent Lodge Program for people with dementia. The Baptist Union, Mission of St James and St John, the Salvation Army and others all provide a variety of community service programs including hostel, nursing home and day care services. Further exchange can occur by attending peer or staff support groups with workers from these other centres (see Appendix B).

Local schools

As already mentioned, school children are a wonderful source of entertainment and fun. The schools are often also willing to lend equipment. (See Chapter 11.)

Community education programs

Older people in residential care should have access to continuing education programs (see Chapter 12 and Appendix E for further details of courses and groups available).

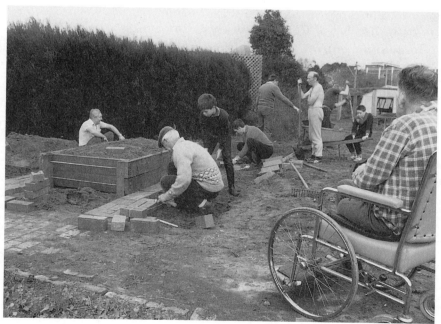

Combining with the local secondary school to build raised garden beds and create a community garden at the rear of the nursing home grounds.

TAFE colleges: Many campuses throughout Australia provide community education courses as well as tertiary courses. Contact the central TAFE office or local campus for details. Some have a special focus for older adults such as the 'Learning for the Less Mobile' program described in Chapter 12.

The Council of Adult Education   a major TAFE provider, offers a broad range of courses for adults and many of them are attended by older people. They also have a special series of subjects for students over 55 years of age. They provide an information and advisory service.

Each State has similar educational bodies with varying titles. In Adelaide and Sydney, it is the Workers' Education Association; in Melbourne, the Council of Adult Education; in Canberra, the Australian National University of Continuing Education Centre. Tasmania has a variety of regional bodies. These groups usually advertise through the newspapers or letterbox drops, so watch out for information and relevant courses.

Information services

There are many information services available, which will help in the development of useful resources and contacts.

Citizens' Advice Bureaus: These centres are available in most cities and can give information about leisure and recreation facilities. The locations of centres are listed in the main body of the telephone directory under the heading of Citizens' Advice Bureaus.

Community Centres: Staff at these centres can direct you to support groups which exist in the local area, and also to neighbourhood groups which some of the residents may have attended in the past.

Commonwealth Department of Sport, Recreation and Tourism produces a number of helpful publications, for example, *Roundup*, which issues information about successful fitness projects, including a focus on older adults (see Appendix A).

State Departments of Sport and Recreation: Within each State department there is a consultancy service which looks at the recreation needs of older adults. This body can be contacted to establish links with other groups and to gain recreation information. Each State produces regular regional news publications which you can use for regular updating of your file. The Victorian department has produced a useful directory of camp facilities suitable for campers in wheelchairs, and they also have a number of videos which provide some stimulating ideas for activities and staff in-service training (see Appendix A).

Commonwealth Government bookshops   sell up-to-date information such as the *Accessibility Guide*, produced by the Commonwealth Department of Sport, Recreation and Tourism. These shops are listed in the telephone directory.

Commonwealth Department of Immigration and Ethnic Affairs and the State **Ethnic Affairs Commission** can direct inquirers to local and regional community groups who will be able to offer advice for national days, give information about entertainers, and link individual residents with cultural groups in the community which the resident may wish to attend.

State Departments of Tourism and **Tourist Bureaus** can offer advice on outings, tours and holidays which are appropriate and accessible for older people. (Refer to your local telephone directory for the relevant office.)

Australian Council on the Ageing (ACOTA) is based in Melbourne and is the only Commonwealth-assisted body concerned with the needs of older Australians. It works to represent the needs of older people with the overall objective of ensuring that, as people grow older, they 'can look forward to a life of dignity, security and one which will enhance and develop their role in society, taking into account their individual economic, social, cultural and medical situations'. ACOTA gathers information about the effectiveness of policies and services affecting older people and presents the needs of older people to governments, service providers and the public. It publishes the *Australian Journal on Ageing* and has a substantial library of relevant books and journals (see Appendix D).

State Councils on the Ageing: Each State has its own representative council which is actively involved in the provision of services for older people. They include advocacy, community education and actual service provision in a large variety of areas. Contact ACOTA for details.

(One such body is the Victorian Council on the Ageing which is based at the same address as ACOTA and has similar objectives. It is involved in advocacy, education, the coordination of service providers, research, information distribution and specific service provision, and has an advisory and counselling service. It has also been instrumental in developing the 'Exercise to Music' training course for leaders of groups of older adults with the Department of Sport and Recreation in Victoria, now being offered through TAFE colleges. The Council has recently developed a weekly talkback program on radio station 3AW, in Melbourne.)

Red Cross Society: State representatives of this society are listed in the telephone directory. The Red Cross is involved in the provision of many recreational and activity programs. They have a large library of books and resource materials which can be borrowed to assist program development and often an advisory service for workers.

Disability information services

There is a wide range of information services which will direct inquirers to the relevant service providers. They may offer information about particular disabilities or about support groups, access, holiday and outing venues and services. They are an excellent starting point for the collection of resource information. Many have computer database services which are regularly updated.

Alzheimer's Society: The Society's aims are:

- to give families and other carers of affected persons an opportunity to assist and encourage one another and to share and discover information regarding the condition of Alzheimer's disease and related disorders
- to educate and inform the public and medical and helping professionals
- to advise government authorities on the needs of the affected persons and their families
- to promote research and seek to improve services for people with Alzheimer's disease and related disorders.

Support groups exist throughout metropolitan and country areas in each State to provide support and information for relatives and carers of people with dementia. Information about the groups can be obtained by contacting your State office, which also acts as an information and referral centre for those who work with people with dementia (see Appendix A for interstate contacts).

Australian Council for Rehabilitation of the Disabled (ACROD) is a national disability information service which can direct inquirers to a large resource of literature, services, self-help groups, and recreation and access information. They produce a number of publications and have an extensive library available for borrowing through the mail (see Appendix A).

Disabled persons information bureaus: This is an up-to-date information resource service which can direct you to relevant self-help groups and organisations to help meet your needs. The title of this service varies in each State (see Appendix A).

This service offers information and assistance in the areas of access, accommodation, home alteration, attendant care, advocacy, employment, education integration, recreational facilities and activities, transport, information on disabilities and self-help group contacts. They have some specific resource information for older people, as well as general information. They will provide excellent information on access to holiday and outing venues, as well as up-to-date details of recreational activities.

Independent living centres (ILC): The ILC is a free advisory service available to anyone in need of information about access or aids for daily living. It displays the full range of aids and equipment which are available, and offers an opportunity for the client to test the suitability of the item. Visits are by appointment only, as the client will be given individual advice from an occupational therapist. The Centre then provides a list of suppliers so that the client can investigate purchasing options (see Appendix A for interstate addresses).

Art and drama resources

If funds allow, the involvement of artistic people can introduce some very stimulating and creative ideas and programs to the centre. Some groups will offer their services free of charge, but others require reasonable payment. In some cases a community arts grant or a trust fund may be prepared to help finance the project.

Local government: There may be a Community Arts Officer in your borough who can assist with art program inquiries.

Senior citizen and local drama groups: There are various groups of older people interested in drama and music who will perform in return for a good afternoon tea and travelling costs. Some offer plays and skits; others, musical items. Your local senior citizen or bowling club may be able to direct you to performers in your region.

Art Centres in capital cities and regional centres often give free or discounted performances for pensioners. These are advertised in the major newspapers.

Colleges of the Arts: There are various groups of artists and schools of art and entertainment throughout Australia whose students may be willing to perform at your centre. However, the students are usually trying to pay their way and may require payment at professional rates to warrant their time.

Many of the colleges or conservatoriums have regular free concerts on campus, in addition to performances at much cheaper rates than commercial productions.

Artists in residence: Some artists are employed to work in various health care centres and run very innovative and positive programs for their clients. Arts Access is one way in which artists can become involved in extended care settings.

Arts Access Society Inc (Vic) is a society committed to providing access to the arts to those groups and individuals disadvantaged by physical, intellectual, emotional or financial conditions. The society links artists with groups or individuals to develop programs which enable people to participate in some form of art.

Arts Access has a particular commitment to establishing pilot and demonstration programs which can be developed and/or replicated by other organisations. They have been involved in a number of programs with older people; drama, writing, movement and cross-generational projects. They are financed by grants from the government and by trusts and donations. It is well worth becoming a member of this society.

Theatre restaurants: Some theatre restaurants will offer entertainment at no cost. This is best arranged by holding a staff or resident dinner at the restaurant, then inviting the performers to call in to the home some time! Well worth it.

Casting agencies can also refer entertainers who may be happy to attend the nursing home.

General resources

Listed below are services and departments which may be able to assist you with information. They can all be found in the telephone directory, usually in the State and local government sections. Some may have slightly different titles from State to State; look in the 'Easy Guide' to government and public services section of the telephone directory if you are not sure of the correct title. Also, the information bureaus listed may be able to give the accurate title and information required for services in your area.

Most of these government and business groups have a public relations department with staff trained to present films and slides and give information about their services. If there is an area in which residents are interested, the groups are usually happy to visit and give a presentation.

Aboriginal Program Exchange
Art Galleries
Association for the Blind (for services and guide dog demonstrations)
Australian Airline Travel Promotion
Australia Day Council
The Board of Works water supply
The Budgerigar Council
Disabled Motorist Association (access information)
Early Retirement Associations
Ethnic Affairs Department
Fire Brigade
Fisheries and Wildlife Department
Forestry Commission
Folk Dancing Society
The Gallery Society
Government Tourist Bureau
Greek Orthodox Community
Hand Weavers and Spinners Guild
Japanese Trade Centre
Lapidary Clubs
Lions Hearing Dog Inc (based in Adelaide)
Metropolitan Research (will give demonstrations and test food products with residents)
National Heart Foundation
National Trust
Police
Railway Institute
Royal Automobile Clubs (accessibility guides)
Royal Historical Society
Royal Horticultural Society (demonstrations, advice and garden experts)
Scottish Board of Highland Dancing
School of Modelling
Senior Citizens Clubs
State Concert Hall (often has special pensioner rate concerts)
Tourist Bureaus (select bureau to suit your national event)

Tapestry Workshops   University Conservatorium
Toast Mistress Clubs   Zoo Visiting Service

Staff development centres

Staff at aged care facilities should have access to courses for professional development. Special expertise is necessary for aged care and staff need the opportunity to keep up-to-date. Staff development is also a necessary morale booster. Many of the Colleges of Advanced Education and Health Sciences offer short or part-time courses for workers. In addition, many of the professional associations run seminars and training courses relevant to aged care.

Mayfield Centre

The Mayfield Centre in Melbourne is the hospital and health services staff training and development body in Victoria. It runs short courses, special projects, extended and certificate courses, and provides consultancy services. This centre is worth mentioning because of its Aged Care Advisory Service and its video package which is available nationally for on-site training and development.

Called 'Activities for Quality of Life in Residential Care', it is a training/advisory package which significantly assists in lifestyle enrichment for residents. The service may be individually presented to meet the particular needs of each nursing home or extended care facility, following on-site discussion. Alternatively, a package program of manuals and self-instructional videotapes is available for purchase (see Appendix B for details).

Their short courses are designed for Carers of Elderly and Disabled Persons, Registered and State Enrolled Nurses, Allied Health Assistants and Therapists Aides, and Supervisors of Domiciliary Care (see Appendix B for the address of the Mayfield Centre). Similar centres in other States are also listed in Appendix B.

Colleges of Health Sciences

Western Australia, New South Wales, Victoria and South Australia each have training campuses which run the various paramedical degree courses. Staff are usually willing to provide an advisory role to help professionals working in the field. They also run a number of postgraduate courses including one in gerontology (see Appendix B).

TAFE Gentle Exercise Training Courses: The Victorian Council on the Ageing (VCOTA) was originally funded to pilot a Gentle Exercise Training Program for workers with older adults. Frankston College of TAFE has established an accredited training course in Gentle Exercise Programs for older adults, and other TAFE colleges will also be running courses. The Australian Council on the Ageing (ACOTA), VCOTA or the Frankston College of TAFE can be contacted for further details.

Creative Art Courses: There are many dance, art, movement and drama, and relaxation (therapy) associations throughout Australia which run short courses for anyone interested. Look around, there may be something which could significantly contribute to your program. They are often good to refresh staff motivation.

Staff support groups

It is most important to become part of a support group with other workers in the field. This will open up a much greater source of information and ideas, as well as offering a way to gain support and encouragement.

Professional associations

Australian Association of Occupational Therapists: There are Australian and State associations of occupational therapists. The AAOT is a member of the World Federation of Occupational Therapists, and produces a quarterly journal which all State members receive. The State associations also produce monthly newsletters which provide valuable information about support groups, seminars and updates on the latest innovations in the field.

These associations have often established specific study groups which meet regularly. If consultancy services are required, the association can direct you to the relevant person. In addition, they often run short training courses for workers in aged care. The State associations can also direct you to the colleges which offer the various staff development courses in that State (see Appendix B).

The Institute of Recreation is the national body for workers with a recreation background — State and regional groups can be contacted through the Institute (see Appendix B).

Australian Council for Health, Physical Education and Recreation, Inc (ACHPER) is a national association for professional people who are committed to promoting healthy lifestyles. Its particular focus is recreation. They have recently begun to focus attention on workers in aged care and are establishing a national resource file of services and centres offering recreational programs to older people in residential care. It will be a valuable resource service. Branches exist in each State and Territory of Australia (see Appendix B).

Other support groups for workers

There are many locally based support groups which grow out of a desire among workers to gain peer support. For example, a group in Melbourne has recently established the 'Older Adults Recreation Network' and another is called 'Leisure Link'. These groups offer support and advocacy for workers in the field. The Department of Sport and Recreation or your professional association in each State can direct you to those groups which work specifically with older adults.

Geriaction　(formerly the Australian Association for Geriatric Nursing Care): Membership is open to anyone with an interest in the care of older people. It seeks to disseminate information through seminars, create awareness of the need for quality, dignity and independence in the lives of older people, lobby governments, and support people who work with or care for older people. It produces a newsletter for members (see Appendix B).

Conclusion

Most resources can be collected with only a small amount of effort. Agencies are usually eager to be of assistance and, if they cannot help directly, will always point you in the direction of someone who can. There tends to be a snowball effect with resources — one source leads to another. And if the entire team at the centre is contributing to the resource collection process, someone, somewhere, will always know somebody who can come up with the answer!

Chapter 10
Volunteers
*with Judy Stanton**

Jock must have been one of our most valuable volunteers. He was a well known character on the bowling club circuit, and had a very special place in his Scottish heart for South Port. Jock was a talented piano accordion player and entertainer and he attended monthly for an afternoon singalong with the residents. He also found time to attend all our special events, and he often brought other club members to form a band and sing for the occasion. This Scottish fellow became true blue Aussie, Irish or French at the drop of a hat! Of course, he was in his element on St Andrew's Day, complete with kilt, when he would make arrangements for a bagpipe player to entertain and pipe in the haggis. His only payment — a glass of scotch whisky!

Every centre needs to find a Jock or two if it can. And don't be surprised if you find one easily through the local bowling or senior citizen clubs.

Volunteers: a link with the community

Volunteers are a crucial part of the team. They have a very significant role to play in working with staff and residents of aged care facilities to create a lively homelike environment. They also ensure that residents maintain strong links with the local community. Volunteers can contribute directly to the quality of life within the centre and also derive great personal benefit from their participation. They add a whole new dimension to the lives of the residents.

The people who choose to become volunteers can fulfil many roles — ones of friendship, companionship, entertainment, and assistance to individual residents and staff, for example. And if volunteers are part of the local community they can be active 'public relations persons' for aged

---

* Judy Stanton was the coordinator of volunteers at South Port Community Nursing Home. She has a background in psychology and a postgraduate diploma in Gerontology.

care, providing important community links and information resources for residents. These roles clearly offer mutual benefit to residents, staff and the volunteers themselves.

It is important to note, however, that their roles need to be clear, their work appreciated and their identity affirmed. They must never become a source of free labour. Instead, they offer a whole new range of services to residents that no other group can give.

Recruitment

The recruitment of volunteers is a sensitive issue and must be guided by a strong sense of the philosophy of the centre and the role of volunteers in the organisation. Volunteers must 'fit in' with the centre — they need to be liked by the residents, to provide a real service, work well alongside staff and link well with each other. The coordinator of volunteers has an active role in promoting this.

To recruit volunteers, the centre needs to offer a broad range of areas of involvement for them in order to ensure that the centre is of 'use' to

A volunteer serves the afternoon tea.

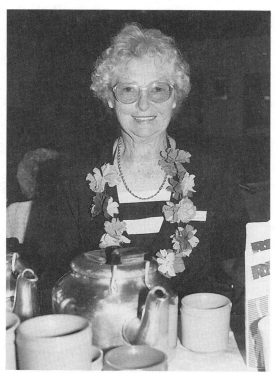

the community. It will then be a place where people from the community can find friendship and chances for work experience, and where they can gain affirmation of their skills.

This is especially important for the spouse, son or daughter who is now living alone since their relative has entered extended care. He or she will often appreciate the opportunity to participate more fully in the life of the centre as it will help to fill the gap left by their relative's departure and to dispel some of the resulting loneliness.

If a variety of areas of involvement are made available, they are more likely to match the breadth of interests and personalities of potential volunteers. As a result, volunteers will reflect, far more, the range of people in the local community. They will offer a wider range of personalities and areas of interest to match those of the residents.

Volunteers come from a variety of sources:

- relatives of residents
- friends of residents
- friends of current volunteers
- friends and family of staff
- members of the community — neighbours, interested people
- service clubs
- school children
- volunteer centres

The need for volunteers can be spread by word of mouth, or by advertising in local shops, newspapers and neighbourhood groups. Other volunteers are usually in touch with local community networks and can spread the word, too. The coordinator of volunteers certainly needs to become a well-established figure in these community networks. She can achieve this by visiting the many centres, speaking to groups and getting to know local identities.

When recruiting volunteers, the coordinator should observe the following characteristics carefully:

- their attitudes towards older people and the way these are expressed and demonstrated
- their motivation for being a volunteer
- how they fit in with the philosophy and attitudes of the organisation

Volunteers working at a nursing home are entering and becoming a part of the residents' home and lives. They must respect this fact, and approach each individual with sensitivity and discretion. Their attitude must be one of being with friends and equals who are valued and important human beings. They must never be patronising.

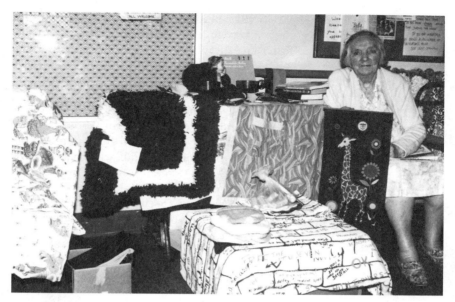

A resident becomes a volunteer as she looks after the residents' stall.

Take all prospective volunteers for a walk through the nursing home, to observe how they interact with people they meet and the comments they make on the experience. This often clearly reflects their attitudes. Ask directly about their motivation for volunteering. Follow this with a detailed description of the range of work available to them and the expectations of them as volunteers within the organisation.

Encourage volunteers to select their own area of participation and time commitment. This will ensure that each person's resources are developed and applied creatively, bringing all-round satisfaction to both volunteer and residents. The minimum time commitment is usually half a day a week — this much is needed to feel a part of the place. However, over-commitment can lead to either burnout or excessive dependency on the nursing home.

Once recruited, volunteers agree to a four-week probation period, during which they can cease involvement or be requested to do so. At the same time, it gives everyone an opportunity to see whether the selected area of involvement suits them.

Supervision from other staff

The coordinator of volunteers can offer considerable supervision and support, but she will not always be available when volunteers are participating in activities at the centre. Other staff will need to offer direction, support and encouragement to the volunteers working with them. The centre should encourage staff to recognise the value of volunteers in the lives of the residents, and foster an attitude among staff of acceptance and encouragement towards volunteers. This can be achieved by in-service training, and by the development of good relationships between the co-ordinator of volunteers, the volunteers themselves and the staff.

Staff must not feel that their employment opportunities are being taken over by volunteers. Volunteers are not a source of cheap labour — they should be seen as as a means of enhancing the lives of the community of people at the centre. Any help they may offer to staff will enable those staff to spend more time chatting with the residents and getting to know them better. Cooperation and communication with unions may be necessary in some areas. The union may want to specify clearly the limits of volunteer involvement. Union members will also need careful education in the value and purpose of volunteer participation, so that everyone is happy to support this involvement.

Support

The coordinator must always be aware of volunteers' levels of satisfaction with their activities, and the possible need to modify their tasks. She must be readily available to answer queries, and she will need to vary her times of attending the centre so as to meet all the volunteers at some stage. Again, other staff will need to offer support and direction as needed.

The number of volunteers involved needs to be monitored so that they can be adequately supervised. There are also important administrative considerations, such as adequate insurance cover, support of staff and unions, and training, when considering how many can be involved, and in what areas.

Volunteers have to grapple with their role in the organisation and they do need to know they are appreciated. The coordinator of volunteers and the other staff at the centre need to be aware of this, and offer both spontaneous and structured signs of appreciation.

A sense of their identity as a group and as part of the organisation is essential to this process. Quarterly meetings of the entire group will enable them to meet each other, make suggestions for improvements, and be kept up-to-date about any changes in the nursing home and its functioning. We give a Christmas party each year just for the volunteers, as a special forum for thanks and as a celebration of their invaluable contribution to the centre.

Areas of involvement

The opportunities for volunteer involvement are as vast as your imagination allows them to be. It is important to use the resources this group

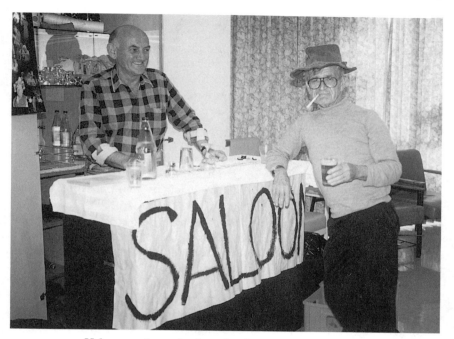

Volunteers keep the beer flowing at a special event.

brings to the situation, as this maximises diversity, affirms their skills and allows people a level of comfort with their involvement. Specific training opportunities may arise, but these should be seen as optional extras rather than necessary for all.

However, the limits of what volunteers can and cannot do must be clearly stated for everyone's safety, and each centre will need to determine its own set of limits. They may include such things as not lifting or transferring residents, the extent of assistance volunteers offer other staff, and careful education on the rights of the residents to privacy and control over their own lives.

Our experience in a community-based nursing home suggests that involving age groups from babies to 80 years plus is a great advantage. Volunteers can assist in all aspects of the daily running of the nursing home — laundry, sewing, bedmaking, administration, driving visitors and residents to and from the centre, morning and afternoon teas, therapy and activities, provision of music, and recreational pursuits. There are many chances just to chat and be with individual residents. Children and babies are a great source of companionship and offer the excuse to participate in fun activities.

Examples of volunteer involvement

Babies become volunteer cuddlers and playmates. Many quite confused residents respond most appropriately and safely with babies. Babies may like to visit for short periods or attend for a number of hours to join in various group activities with their mothers. They are a great source of pleasure and entertainment.

Children also offer a special kind of companionship and friendship. They may be children of staff, or relatives of residents, or neighbours from the local area. They may like to attend just to chat with people or to join in activities. Children can have a significant effect on the atmosphere of many group activities. A lively exchange of laughter and chatting usually results (see Chapter 11).

Companions: Some volunteers may attend simply to be with certain residents they find they get on well with. Such volunteers can be of any age. We had a very special volunteer, a woman who was between jobs and had a sensitive and caring attitude towards a very confused and disabled resident. She would sit and talk quietly and gently stroke the resident's hand, offering a form of companionship that few others had the time and skills to offer. The volunteer gained satisfaction from seeing slight changes in the light and expression of the resident's eyes — she saw them as efforts to show appreciation for her special care.

This volunteer had special skills and patience which few of us can match. However, many volunteers can form natural friendships with residents who may not be quite so severely disabled. Invariably, every volunteer who attends to do a particular task will develop friendships with at least a few of the residents. Their value to the home for this reason alone is immeasurable.

Administration: Volunteers can assist with typing, answer the telephone, and relieve staff from the reception area during breaks. Volunteers often enjoy working in this central position.

Driving: Volunteer drivers can bring in relatives, take residents to visit relatives, or shopping, help with outings, and take residents to regular classes.

Activity assistants: Volunteers can assist with all the weekly activities described in Chapter 4. As well as being extra help, they create a more social and convivial atmosphere which encourages residents to join in.

Sewing: This may include attaching name labels to clothing, repairing clothes, finishing crafts, or making items to sell at the residents' stall or fete.

Residents' stall: In this case the residents become volunteers. The stall can be supervised by a team of residents and sell a variety of items made by the residents themselves, or donated by relatives and friends. The stall

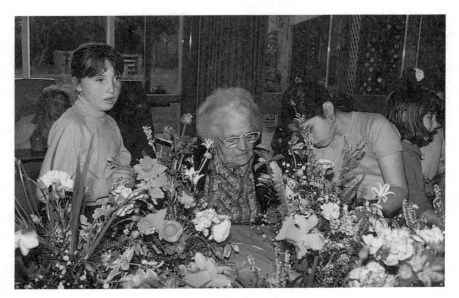

Children can also be volunteers.

is best situated in the entrance hall, so 'passerbuyers' will be tempted. Raffles can also be run from this vantage point. Volunteers can help by contributing stock. Very little staff involvement is required.

Art gallery: With the help of volunteers, invite local artists to display their work for sale in the entrance area and corridors of the home. The paintings should be changed regularly. This provides interest for the residents and also another avenue through which to invite the community into the home.

Club nights: Volunteers and evening staff may like to get together with residents once a fortnight for a club night. The activity can vary with the requests of the residents, but might include viewing a video or film, or a card night. Residents stay up later than usual and invite friends or relatives to join them in these activities. Relatives and friends bring in supper. These events help to normalise sleep patterns, as there is a tendency for nursing home residents to go to bed early, at an age when the need for sleep is significantly reduced.

Groups led by volunteers

Volunteers are essential to the success of an activities program. Mostly, they prefer to help the activity coordinator to run groups, yet a few can be found who have the personal resources and abilities to run their own groups. A little advertising and detective work is needed to discover those volunteers who already have skills and interests which enable them to lead groups themselves. They may like to run them alone or with the assistance of other volunteers and staff. Some may develop confidence over time, and move from group assistant to leader with a little support and encouragement.

What follows is a sample of the groups we have had run by volunteers. The particular talents of your own volunteers will determine the nature of the groups which can be run.

Quizzes: A local resident from the community who ran quizzes for the senior citizen and service groups came in to run them for residents. He was particularly skilled, having a greater understanding of the interests and memories of an older group of people. He planned and ran the group without assistance.

Travelogue Group: We were fortunate to find a volunteer with experience as a tour guide, and she led discussions about countries of the world. About 6 to 8 residents gathered in a quiet room to hear about the lifestyles of other cultures, see souvenirs and clothing, pass round photographs, and hear anecdotes of the travels. It was a very popular group.

Stamp Group: A small group of residents met weekly to trim stamps from envelopes, then sort and package the stamps. The volunteer organised this group completely, arranging for local business and councils to save their envelopes and to deliver them to the home. He also arranged the sale of stamps to a dealer. The proceeds were used in whatever way the group chose, for the benefit of the home or for some other charity.

Singalongs: A musical volunteer can usually be found to run singalongs. A pianist may like to attend weekly to play for half an hour before lunch, for example. Our greatest success was our monthly visit from Jock, a Scottish piano accordion player. Volunteers for singalongs need to have a good knowledge of songs appropriate to the age of the residents. Such people can usually be found at the local service clubs.

Conclusion

Volunteers are the key to bringing the local community into the nursing home, enabling the home to become a natural part of the neighbourhood. Volunteers need to feel valued members of the team and the centre must offer them opportunities for development and personal benefit. A great community exchange results and the lives of both residents and volunteers are significantly enriched.

Chapter 11
Children and School Involvement

with Judy Stanton

Jean was a delightful but confused resident; very bright, artistic, but often lost in the world of her past, which had been colourful and exciting, far more stimulating than her present circumstances. Everyone said she had no recent memory, which contributed to her confusion.

However, she participated fully in the program, particularly enjoying her contact with children. She rarely, if ever, knew the names of the staff who worked with her, and she often thought she was staying in a motel, or on board a ship to India. The only people she did recognise by name were her family.

Yet children and babies had a special impact on her. When my daughter Philippa was only a few months old, I took her with me to South Port for a few hours each week. After Jean had spent a short time cuddling Philippa and getting to know her, every time we met, she would say: 'Let me see the baby. It's Philippa, isn't it?'

Children

Everyone acknowledges the special relationship which so often occurs between the very old and the very young; there seems to be a special kind of magic which exists just between these two age groups. It is a great tragedy if the extended care environment prevents these groups from getting together. Children must be encouraged to attend the centre and to feel at home and at ease within this unusual environment.

Children of all ages play a very significant role in the lives of older people. In a situation where residents often feel incapable of contributing to the well-being of others, children offer a focus for their care and interest. Consistently, confused people brighten at the sight of a baby and respond in a very appropriate manner. Staff, volunteers and relatives can all be encouraged to bring their children in on a regular basis. However, structured programs with schools, creche and playgroups help to increase the frequency and predictability of contacts with the younger generation.

Involvement with school and creche groups gives residents an opportunity

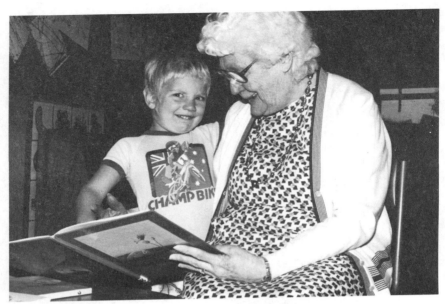

Story time at the creche.

to link in with the activities of the local community in a very positive way. They have the chance to give of themselves and develop a greater sense of purpose in their lives. It is another way in which life in a nursing home can be full of surprises and new experiences for its residents despite their age, disabilities and living environment.

Playgroups

Staff, neighbours, and relatives can bring their toddlers for a weekly playgroup at the home. Residents who would like to participate in the playgroup program can do so; others simply enjoy watching the children play nearby. This type of group can become the high point of the week for those residents who particularly enjoy the company of children.

Equipment: A toy library can supply most toys, while mothers can bring in others.

Staff: After the initial establishment of the group, it may become self-directive and only need assistance to set itself up each week.

Time: 1–2 hours is usually plenty.

Creche assistants

A small group of residents can visit the local creche each week to help the children in their activities. It creates a wonderful exchange. The children

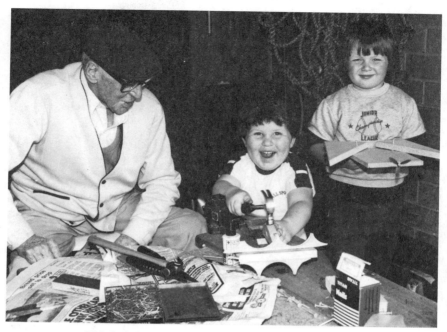

Helping the children with their construction work.

love their new friends, and often contribute to the special events back at the home.

Equipment: Car or bus transport.

Staff: One staff member, a volunteer driver and assistants.

Time: The whole trip will take about 2 hours.

Primary school groups

A class from a local school can be invited to attend weekly. The teacher will usually decide to divide the class into smaller groups which attend, say, for a period of 6 weeks. Ten to 12 residents are then matched with as many children. The teacher may like to involve the children in activities at school which can be brought to share with residents. Usually a child is matched with a resident, to encourage them to develop a friendship over the time. They meet in the lounge where a terrific buzz develops which everyone can enjoy.

Many children do not experience a sense of the extended family as they did in the past and have little contact with older people. The nursing home can offer them grandparent figures who take a special interest in them and help them to gain a broader view of life and history. The

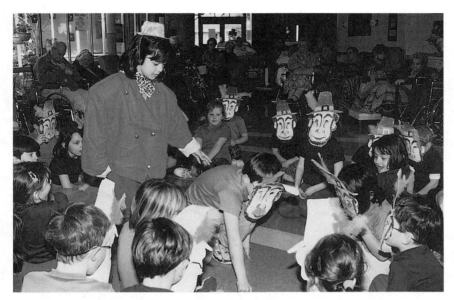

Primary school children act out a leprechaun play for St Patrick's Day.

children offer the residents friendship, an excuse for lively activity, and an opportunity to think beyond themselves and their own needs.

Time: The sessions last about 45 minutes unless a special activity is planned. The session just before lunch is best as it allows some extension of time if needed.

Staff: The school teacher can usually offer a whole new spectrum of ideas and activities for these sessions, if he or she is enthusiastic and committed to the idea. The activity coordinator and teacher arrange the program together. Other volunteers are helpful but not essential.

Activity ideas could include discussions at school on ageing and mutual areas of interest to help prepare the children for the sessions. Children may have reading practice with their resident, or draw pictures, make cards and displays for the centre. They may sing or perform plays and concerts. The students may like to bring in their current school projects to show to their resident. The centre can organise games, cooking, ice-cream making and parties for the children. Some residents may like to attend the school to help with its reading program.

High school groups

Tutorship program

A tutorship program can be developed, which matches selected residents with students from a local high school who may have learning difficulties.

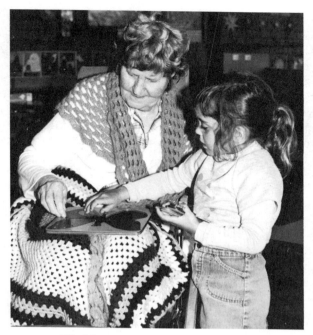

Working together to solve a puzzle.

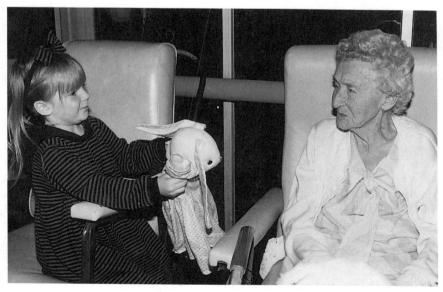

Sharing a special moment.

If students are encouraged to attend the centre each week over a number of years, strong friendships develop. This is a particularly valuable program as it creates an exchange between two very different generations where both groups gain a great deal from each other.

Apart from increased literacy and social skills, the students have the opportunity to learn some history in an informal way. In addition, many will be meeting older people for the first time. One student, describing his relationship with his tutor, said he had found someone he could tell his problems to. He found it so much easier to develop a trusting relationship with this older person than with his schoolmates.

The confidence and self-esteem of the participants increases significantly as a result of these projects. Strong friendships are established and increased knowledge across generations is gained.

Four to six students with specific learning needs can attend each week to read and practise conversational skills with an individually matched tutor (resident). Two different groups may like to attend each week. Together the tutor and student choose and complete a project of mutual benefit. For example, a student may develop a written history of the resident's life, and present it in booklet form to the tutor at the end of the semester. Others may work on a woodwork, garden, cooking or craft project.

Projects might include:

- 'My Life Story' — we had the delightful combination of a Vietnamese student learning English interviewing a 93-year-old woman with a broad Lancashire accent.
- 'Changes I Have Seen in my Lifetime' — comments by a 91-year-old juxtaposed with those of a 13-year-old.
- 'My Life in the Army' — a school cadet talks with an 85-year-old about his army experiences.
- 'Changes in the Local Area' — this covered interviews about the resident's life and a drive around the area, comparing photographs and reminiscing.
- Writing poetry together.

Or all of the above can be compiled into one large book. Encourage students to keep a journal of their visits, from which to collect anecdotes and experiences. Other discussion ideas can include career options, mutual interest topics such as sport, or childhood memories of being a rebel. Others may have reading practice, bringing in a library book to read with a resident. Here the resident needs to know how to correct mistakes sensitively.

Thorough preparation, ongoing supervision and monitoring of this program and its participants is essential to its success. The coordinator of

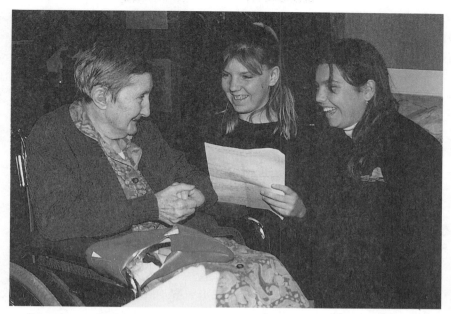

Secondary school students present their 'Life Story' project to their tutor.

volunteers and the school teachers work together to oversee the program. A video called 'Really Good Friends' has been made about such a program. It is available for hire or purchase, with an accompanying booklet (see Appendix C).

Other students from the school may also ask to visit residents to interview them as part of their local history projects.

Staff: Usually 1 or 2 remedial teachers will supervise 4–6 students. One centre staff member will need to assist in the initial establishment of the project and offer continued support and encouragement. However, at most times, the tutor and student will be able to work together unsupervised.

Time: Usually 1 hour is sufficient for each session.

School volunteer program

The community liaison teacher of the local high school can be contacted and arrangements made to bring 4–6 students each week, as part of their community services program. The students may wish to make a weekly commitment to carry out specific activities at the centre. Tasks can include distributing morning tea or water jugs, making beds, playing cards or games and organising the weekly bingo game. The students may also like to provide the prizes through fundraising. The end result is that many of these students will develop friendships with residents while visiting.

Staff: After the initial establishment of the projects, the school teacher can supervise the sessions, while the activity coordinator or coordinator of volunteers may need only to offer support, encouragement and some time together with the teacher to exchange ideas.

Extended involvement

With all these school programs, many exchange activities can develop between students and residents.

- Residents may attend the school for special functions, such as celebratory days and parties.
- The students may help with preparations for special events.
- Students may perform excerpts from their school concerts, or plan a concert specifically for the home. The concerts can include rap dancing, international dancing, singing and skits.
- Students may also attend to help run the movement to music sessions.
- Residents can regularly attend the school for art classes.
- The students can be invited to go on holidays with the residents.
- Students may drop in after school or during their holidays to visit.

Work experience students

Secondary school students may like to do their work experience placements at the nursing home. There are many varied employment opportunities at most aged care facilities. Depending on their interests, students could attend to observe and assist therapists, recreation staff, nurses, domestic, administrative or gardening departments. Occasionally, lasting relationships will develop between students and residents.

The community liaison teacher is a great resource person for ideas and community projects which link residents and students. She will be aware of other service projects and needs in the community which the residents and students may be able to contribute to together.

Tertiary students

Students from the various professional groups should be encouraged to have placements in aged care facilities. Many students do not realise the potential of working with older people and have a fairly negative attitude towards it. They need the opportunity to observe innovative, positive centres in action. This has two effects: it educates students and broadens their attitudes to working with older adults, and it encourages more professionals to make a deliberate choice to work in the field after graduation.

There must be adequate supervision of the students by the relevant professional group. Students will need plenty of time to observe activities and discuss programs with staff and residents, and then the opportunity to carry out their own activities. Adequate time must be allowed for feedback and discussion. Occupational therapy, nursing and recreation students can all gain a great deal from such specialised experience, assuming the relevant staff are working in the centre.

There is mutual benefit in working with tertiary students. Not only do they learn more about the ageing population, but they bring with them new ideas and a fresh approach which can contribute significantly to the lives of the residents.

At one centre where a recreation officer is the activity coordinator, four recreation students attended to run a bush dance for the residents. Before the day they devised special steps for wheelchair users, which involved interaction between wheelchair user and pusher, and between wheelchair users. No one was restricted from participating. They used taped bush dance music and included all the usual, very active, bush dances. The noise and laughter clearly indicated that the session was a great success. This kind of event would be very difficult for one activity staff member to organise. The students brought to the centre the new idea and the people power to carry it out.

Conclusion

Programs which link students and older adults are particularly worthwhile. A special attraction really does seem to exist between the older and younger generations. Lasting friendships can develop, and a whole new range of activities and areas of involvement appears. Every centre should ensure that residents, children and young people have many opportunities to meet and enjoy each other's company.

Chapter 12
Community Education Programs

Four people from South Port attend the 'Learning for the Less Mobile' (LLM) Armchair Travel sessions held each Monday at the local senior citizens club. Each week a different speaker talks about his or her travels and experiences overseas. Guest speakers have included local identities, tour guides, professional public speakers and a nurse who happens to be the LLM bus driver and has visited Papua New Guinea.

There is much anticipation as the group prepares to leave for the session. In Enid's room there is a flurry of activity as she selects the right outfit and takes extra care to ensure her makeup and hair are just right. Mary doesn't quite remember what the topic will be today. She enjoyed last week's session immensely and chatted brightly about it for the next day or so. She rarely remembers anything beyond that, but it is still worth it for the pleasure she gains.

George and Bob are organising a 'tour' of their own! After an especially interesting presentation about Mongolia, George said to the others: 'I've never been to Mongolia, let's arrange a holiday there.' Bob and Lyn (the nurse/bus driver) agreed to go with him. The next week's talk was about China. 'While we're going to Mongolia, how about we stop over in China on the way?' Bob and Lyn agreed. But the following week when George also added Papua New Guinea to the itinerary, Bob withdrew from that leg of the journey; he reckoned it was much too humid there!

The group finds out at the end of each session where they will be travelling to the following week, so there is much anticipation as everyone plans ahead for the next trip. As they board the bus, the standard joke is: 'Have we all got our passports? Where are we off to today?'

On return home, there is a queue of residents and staff waiting to ask about the trip, and there is always something interesting to tell them. One speaker described the time she was given the honour of carrying the frozen excrement of a rare mountain animal. Unsure what to do with it, and eager not to offend, she pocketed the prized discovery. As they moved on in search of the beast itself, her agitation increased as the item gradually defrosted in its cozy new home. The group had a great time relating this story to others when they returned to the centre.

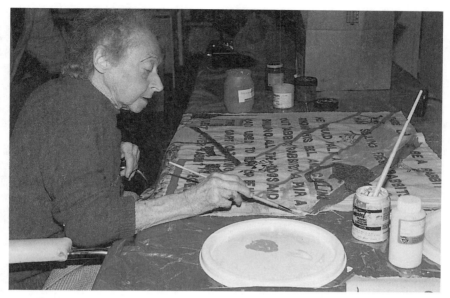

Community Art classes open up opportunities for creative expression.

These anecdotes give just a glimpse of the new experiences, knowledge and pleasures that these people are gaining as they attend the program.

An intellectual challenge

Regardless of the accommodation needs of older people, their need to exercise choice and control over their lives will mean, for some, the opportunity to be involved in further education. Many older people desire some form of intellectual challenge, but most traditional educational facilities do not meet the varied needs of older people seeking further education.

Fortunately, community-based programs designed for older people are being developed, and they play a very important role in the development of a comprehensive activity program. As the policy statement of the Council of Adult Education (CAE) says: 'Education is one means of encouraging a development approach to later life, enhancing the self-esteem, dignity and independence of older persons.'

Community education programs

This chapter will look at some community education programs which are available to older people both in the community and in extended care settings. A description of the program at Grace McKellar House in Geelong provides one example of their value.

Some of the material in this chapter is drawn from a report by Heather Beaton entitled *Learning in the Later Years. A Study about Older Persons Learning.*[1] The report acts as a handbook for organisations wishing to establish educational opportunities for older people. It is available through the Hawthorn Community Education Centre and TAFE (see Appendix E) and describes three quite different programs being run by the Centre. It also looks at educational issues, such as the motivation for study in later years, the delivery and programming of material, the use of volunteers and technical aids to learning.

The report lists, with a brief description, educational projects which exist throughout Australia, and some programs in Europe, Canada and America. It provides a good outline of the potential variety for educational programs. Australian educational centres are listed in Appendix E.

Underlying principles

The important principles which must underpin community education programs include:

- Participants should play a key role in the planning and development of the courses.
- Participants attend to enjoy learning with others. They are not usually looking for assessment or intense lecturing programs.
- Teachers should work alongside the students, creating an atmosphere of shared team learning. The traditional classroom approach of authoritative teacher and passive students is certainly not appropriate.
- The learning process should be creative, including displays of artefacts and objects for discussion, outings, and recreational activities such as singing, exercises and word games.
- The classes should be held at an accessible venue which is light and attractive.

It has generally been found that for older participants the three Cs of formal educations — Credentials, Career and Curriculum — are of no concern to them. They seek a different set of three Cs: Community, Companionship and Comprehension.[1] They want to be part of a community of learners, who all enjoy learning; to meet new people and share new experiences; to acquire an understanding of new knowledge which enriches life.

Hawthorn Community Education Centre has been the brains behind three programs which continue to be successful in Melbourne. They are:

- the 'Learning for the Less Mobile' program
- correspondence course for housebound people
- the University of the Third Age program (U3A)

All three work on a strong consultative model which reflects the principles listed above; in each case the students, volunteers and tutors have designed the programs together.[1]

Learning for the Less Mobile (LLM)

LLM is a program which provides learning groups, film and theatre outings, and other activities for people who are unable to attend conventional classes and tours. This may be due to lack of suitable transport or because many conventional programs do not cater for those with some frailty or disability. Many of the people who participate come from local nursing homes and hostels. The multi-purpose taxi system and community buses are used for transport.

Linking into the network of community health workers and local aged care facilities, networking with various neighbourhood and service groups, and advertising in the local paper all help students and tutors to find each other. Many of the programs are organised by staff from local TAFE colleges.

In some cases the tutors are paid through various sources of community funding, particularly TAFE and other voluntary, adult learning funding organisations. The tutors are assisted by volunteers who play an important part in this program; they are respected as workers and given adequate first-hand 'apprenticeship' training.

Classes vary in nature. There may be a discussion group, a forum for guest speakers, a current affairs and politics group, local history or women in history, poetry and nostalgia, television appreciation, travel groups, or well-being, health and safety classes. Each group is usually led by a tutor in conjunction with 2 volunteers and may have up to 15 participants.

The session usually includes afternoon tea, and a very positive social atmosphere is developed. The cross-section of people from nursing homes, hostels and the local community enjoy the chance to get together.

The aims of the project are:

- to increase learning opportunities for people with limited mobility due to physical and/or social factors
- to provide the opportunity for people to continue to develop socially, emotionally and intellectually through learning
- to allow people to gain greater control over their lives, through the learning experience
- to provide the opportunity for integration and participation in community activities wherever possible, e.g. oral histories, or writing projects with schools
- to discriminate positively in favour of activities and programs that will enhance skill development and the initiation of new community activities

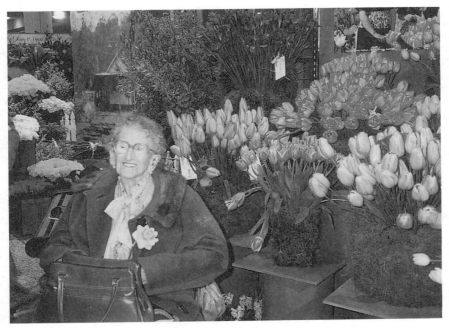

Being part of a garden club means visiting during Garden Week.

- to increase community awareness and promote positive attitudes towards ageing, people with disabilities, and life-long learning[1]

The LLM model is an excellent one for the provision of further education for older people. To quote the Centre's report:

> 'The underpinning philosophy of LLM is one of normalisation, integration and self-determination. Education is a commodity highly valued in our society and should be accessible to everyone. The program offers participants access to decision-making because they determine what they want to learn, in what style, and are encouraged to speak up about their concerns and opinions.'

Correspondence Course for Housebound People

This is a national program, based at Hawthorn Community Education Centre, designed to develop the creative writing skills of its participants.

The underlying philosophies of this program are similar to those mentioned above. It aims to provide those who have limited opportunity to attend classes in the community, due to disability or geographical isolation, with the chance to develop their interest in creative writing.

The course is open to any housebound person of any age in Australia. The focus of the writing activities is on the unique life experience of the individual. Some topics included in the course are:

- childhood
- my background
- events and people that have shaped my life
- change
- myself
- letters and diaries

The course is not designed to train students to become professional writers, but to develop skills in writing for pleasure. Each month the writers receive an assignment, which they complete and return for comment by volunteer encouragers; it is then returned promptly to the writer. A telephone consultation service is available day and evening, 7 days a week, for writers who wish to ask advice or discuss their work.

In its first year, the project was funded by an establishment grant from the Commonwealth Department of Health. It has continued with trust, TAFE and municipal council funding.

University for the Third Age (U3A)

The U3A is a movement which began in France. It is a self-help organisation of older persons who provide their own classes, and operates on similar principles to those already described.

The term 'university' is used as a description of a house of learning. Some TAFE campuses and other college venues are used, but many other venues are also quite appropriate. The 'third age' describes those who are no longer in the workforce, usually those 60 and over, although younger students are usually welcome.

Each campus is autonomous — there is no central organising body. Hence management is styled on the resources and philosophies of each campus. All funding is from membership fees; there are no government subsidies or grants to U3A. Costs are kept to a minimum because of the voluntary nature of the program.

Tutors, students and organisers are all volunteers. Subjects vary along the full spectrum of both academic and general interest — from cell biology to car maintenance — according to the resources of each campus. Tutors in U3A do not need to be accredited teachers. They are usually people with past experience in a certain field who enjoy sharing their knowledge with others. Again, students and tutors share actively in the planning and direction of the courses. Tutors have their own style of teaching; some set homework, others do not.[1]

To demonstrate how the university works, I include here a summary of the U3A program in operation at Grace McKellar House in Geelong.

Grace McKellar is a large institution which faces many structural and administrative difficulties that smaller settings often do not have. Despite this, many activities similar to those described in this book have been successfully applied to this larger setting. The U3A program is perhaps the most innovative activity in operation at present. Glenn Krusic-Golub, the coordinator of activities and volunteers at Grace McKellar, provided the following information.

U3A: Why at Grace McKellar?

Many academic facilities now run a wide variety of courses for the third age, and U3A also has links with the Council for Adult Education. Grace McKellar tapped into these programs, yet found that many of the courses were held in buildings inaccessible to frail older people. It decided to offer its facilities to the third age program as a community campus. The aim was to bring people from both the home itself and the local community together to study topics of mutual interest. The teachers are often volunteers with a special interest or previous professional training.

Meeting differing interests

Not all residents of aged care facilities are interested in craft work or physically capable of joining in active pursuits. However, many do have very lively minds that crave stimulation and new challenges. The introduction of the U3A concept has been received with great enthusiasm by these people. In addition to the personal benefits which each participant experiences in the stimulating and challenging learning environment, the residents often establish new friendships with people from the local community, visiting each other for lunch or a cup of tea.

The classes running at Grace McKellar House include the following.

Art

Venue: Coffee shop, recreation room, or other light airy room.

Equipment: Painting and drawing materials; easels or tables.

Group size: 9–10 students.

Staff: In this case a retired man from the community who loves art.

Time allowance: 9am to 3pm once a week. Tea and coffee are provided; students bring a cut lunch.

Level of participation: This depends entirely on the capabilities of each participant and their commitment to the subject. There really are no limits: a severely disabled person with limited movement in only one hand completed 5 pictures with assistance from the tutor. (Many of the students' paintings were sold to the public on Open Day.)

Value: The overall sense of achievement, social interaction and the feeling of 'being capable' cannot be valued too highly.

Australian history

Venue: Comfortable attractive room, free of distractions.
Equipment: Overhead projector.
Group size: 4–8 students.
Staff: Retired Minister of Religion who has studied and taught history.
Time allowance: 1½ hour session once a week.

Some members have disabilities such as hearing and speech impairments, but much visual material is used, including large pictorial books, and everyone participates actively in the group. One 90-year-old resident, with very restricted movement, is delighted that at long last she has been recognised as having a very active mind. She had not been able to dress herself for over 6 months but, because she was anxious not to be late for the class, she sat on her bed and dressed herself completely, except for tying her shoelaces. The sense of achievement and the motivation behind her attempt is indicative of the mental stimulation the residents have gained from their classes.

Projects: They have twice travelled to the State Offices to study the 'Early Geelong' mural, and had lunch on the top floor of the same building while discussing the mural.

Armchair travel

Venue: Quiet, comfortable room that can be darkened.
Equipment: Slide projector and slides.
Group size: Up to 16 students.
Staff: Retired travel agent.
Time allowance: 1½ hour session once a week.

Level of participation: Students watch slides of the country they are studying, while the tutor tells them about its history and culture.

Value: It could be argued that some of the residents would not gain much, just sitting in a wheelchair watching. But the feedback from nursing staff shows that, at meal times, not only do these residents talk about the country they are studying but that there is much greater stimulation and interest in their conversation generally. This adds to their overall sense of well-being and achievement.

Two other classes about to begin are 'Creative Writing' and 'Introduction to Computers'.

The greatest advantage of using Grace McKellar House as a campus, of course, is that all the facilities are geared for older and disabled residents. Medical attention is near at hand and everything is accessible by wheelchair. The place is buzzing with other activity and they don't feel alone, as they often do in a large CAE building, occupied by much younger people.

All this adds to the students' sense of security and well-being and it also allows the community to view Grace McKellar House in a different light; it becomes a place for learning and living rather than an 'old people's home'.

Television University Studies

In Australia, on ABC Television the *Open Learning Program* provides material for university study each morning at 6am and 7.30am. It covers subjects such as Anthropology, Accounting, Languages, Mathematics, Sciences, History and so on. Study material is then available for students to complete course requirements. This material can be a good resource for U3A and other educational activities.

Conclusion

To meet the varied needs of participants, an activity program should include the opportunity for further learning for those who are interested. The learning needs of older adults are different, but there are many educational services now offering specialised programs for older adults. There is also the potential for exciting 'home-grown' educational initiatives to develop. If these are used to the full, the resources and opportunities for residents are increased immensely.

Reference

1. Beaton H. *Learning in the Later Years. A Study about Older Persons Learning.* TAFE Victoria, 1986. Copyright material used with permission from TAFE VIC. A useful guide for those wanting to tap into existing programs or develop new ones themselves.

Chapter 13
Constructive Visiting
by Kay Dannatt (Waldron)*

Many relatives and friends find it difficult to maintain regular visits to someone resident in aged care for long periods. Some find the unfamiliar environment threatening, others simply run out of things to do and talk about. Others do not fully understand how to 'fit in' with the life of the centre, and feel quite uncomfortable and out of place. Constructive visiting is an approach that ensures residents receive regular visits from their close friends and relatives. It helps both residents and visitors to enjoy the visits and makes visitors feel they have a valuable contribution to make to the lives of the residents.

Studies have shown that where residents in institutions can predict and control visits from friends and relatives, their physical and psychological well-being improves.[1] So constructive visiting also involves finding out from residents which visitors they like to receive, when and how often.

Program structure

The constructive visiting program works at 4 levels:

1. **Staff:** The program is geared towards ensuring that staff see visitors as essential to the care and well-being of residents.

2. **Early intervention:** Efforts are made to assist family and friends in their visiting soon after the admission of their relative. The initial family interview is used to encourage creative visiting and the subsequent 'get-togethers' aim to foster communication and cooperation between staff and visitors.

3. **Education:** The family interview, the get-together, the video and visiting handout are all geared towards educating visitors about the important role they play, and showing them how to make their visits worthwhile.

---

* Kay Dannatt was formerly Chief Occupational Therapist at Alexander Hospital, Castlemaine, Victoria.

They are designed to make sure everyone enjoys the visits and the visitors want to return.

4. **Regular follow-up:** All staff are encouraged to observe visiting patterns, and to encourage and help visitors to make the most of the time with their resident.

Features of the program

The get-together: A structured program to facilitate communication between visitors and staff.

Visitor file: A file is developed of each resident's key relatives and friends so that the appropriate people can be invited to events and outings.

Formal invitations: Individual invitations are sent out for some special events.

The visiting handout: A brochure developed specifically for your centre which gives information and helpful hints for making visits more pleasurable.

The video: Where possible, a personalised video of the centre, providing relevant information of value to visitors.

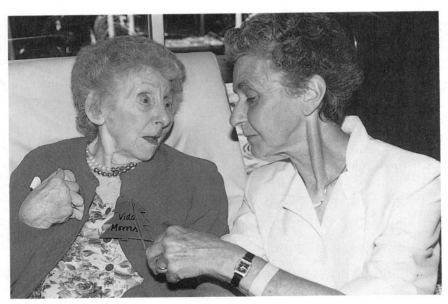

If there is a lot happening at the home there is always something to tell relatives when they visit.

Kay Dannatt describes below a visiting program that she developed. It is designed to encourage relatives and friends to participate more fully in the lives of residents, thus making visits more enjoyable for everyone.

Aims of the program

- to encourage more people to visit their relative or friend
- to emphasise the importance to residents of the continuing support of their visitors
- to make every effort to ensure visitors feel welcome, needed and a part of the centre
- to help visitors with difficulties in visiting (particularly where communication is made difficult by a specific form of disability, such as a speech disorder)
- to encourage visiting which is more meaningful and rewarding for both residents and visitors
- to encourage residents to take an active role in planning the timing and regularity of their visits

Achieving the aims

Staff education

To foster a welcoming atmosphere for visitors, staff education is essential. Staff must recognise that they work in the 'home' of each resident and that relatives and friends are an important part of a person's life and 'home'. Visitors perhaps have a greater right to be with residents than paid staff do, and their visits should not be disrupted unnecessarily. Work routines must be seen as secondary to the main aim of creating a homelike environment for each resident.

Visitors often feel out of place, in the way, interfering or unwelcome; they may also behave as if they were visiting a sick patient rather than their relative at home. All staff should realise the importance of visitors to the well-being or recovery of residents, as well as to their quality of life, and work towards making visitors feel at home in the centre.

Such education can be achieved through seminars, films, discussions and training, whereby attitudes towards visitors can be improved. The aim of the sessions should be to create an openness towards visitors among the staff. Encourage staff to work towards fulfilling these aims:

- To encourage visitors to feel a part of the team of people who seek to make the centre a home for each person in residence.
- To involve visitors and their relatives in the various activities of the centre. This 'normalises' visiting, by re-establishing normal everyday

opportunities for people to do those things together that they may have done in the past. As a result, any sense of visiting a sick person in hospital is dispelled.

- To keep visitors well informed about activities through advertising and invitations.
- To set up more appropriate visiting areas which allow for privacy and have a pleasant atmosphere. Inform visitors of how they can use the various suitable areas (e.g. outdoor sitting areas).

Relative Orientation Program

An intensive Relative Orientation Program should be established where the new resident's relatives are invited to meet key staff to discuss the general principles and activities of the centre. The staff attending the meeting will place particular emphasis on the important role of the visitor.

All close relatives and friends should be involved in the visiting program. Careful homework may be needed by staff to ensure that appropriate relatives are invited to functions, to avoid inviting a feuding relative to attend while neglecting to ask a lifelong friend. A comprehensive list should be developed; close relatives should be able to give information about friends if some residents are unable to do so themselves.

The importance of the visiting program may need to be reinforced at a later date by following up and confirming the information given at the initial orientation sessions.

Routine initial meeting: This meeting, where relatives are introduced to the centre, is a good place to start orienting each person to their new role as 'visitor'. The staff member conducting the meeting can emphasise the important role they have to play in the life of their relative who is entering the centre. At this meeting relatives and friends should be invited to attend a get-together where they will meet the team of people involved in the care of the resident.

The get-together can occur monthly or quarterly, depending on the size of the centre, and covers all new admissions in that period. All recently admitted residents, their friends and relatives, and the staff who will most often be involved in the care of these residents are invited to attend.

The get-together includes:

- The initial welcome and encouragement of visitors. A brief presentation should seek to influence visitors' attitudes and patterns of visiting, particularly at this time when they most need extra support and guidance (but do avoid long speeches).
- A film or video (preferably made by the centre) which clearly explains the various services, assistance and facilities available to visitors. Films create discussion, provoke questions and encourage greater attendance

at the get-together. Other videos and films can also be used here as stimulus material. A school or college could be invited to assist in making the video. (See Appendix C.)

- Afternoon tea to encourage attendance and create a more welcoming atmosphere.
- Handing out the 'Visiting' leaflet and any other relevant information about visiting, activities or the centre.
- Encouraging visitors to approach members of staff in the future; this will be made easier by meeting the staff at the get-together.
- Where necessary, arranging follow-up meetings, e.g. with a speech therapist, if more specific information about the resident's communication difficulties is required; or with the occupational therapist about the resident's level of independence and preferred leisure activities.

This process will encourage an interdisciplinary team approach to visitors, where all staff from every department of the centre work together with the visitors to create a homelike environment for the residents. It is important to emphasise that the visitor is a key member of the team of carers. Another important aim is to keep visitors well-informed about all the various aspects of the life of the home.

Visitor file

Continuing communication should offer up-to-date information to visitors, particularly where their involvement in activities is invited. This will contribute significantly to the maintenance of regular visiting. It is best achieved by talking with each resident to determine who should visit, when and how often. (Where necessary, other close relatives may need to supplement this information.) A mailing list of all close relatives and friends can then be developed for each resident, to ensure that the right people receive invitations to special events.

Information can also be disseminated through a weekly program sheet, indicating the various activities that will occur during the coming week. The sheet can be displayed in the centre. Posters advertising other special events can also be displayed around the centre and on local community and service club notice boards.

The interdisciplinary team should follow up, review and monitor the visiting for each resident in an organised and ongoing manner. For example, a staff member may notice that the frequency of visits is declining for a particular resident. The visitors can be approached informally and encouraged to resume attendance; the staff member should also offer support and assistance to ensure the visits become more pleasurable for everyone. Further guidance may be required long after the settling-in period, particularly if the resident's condition alters.

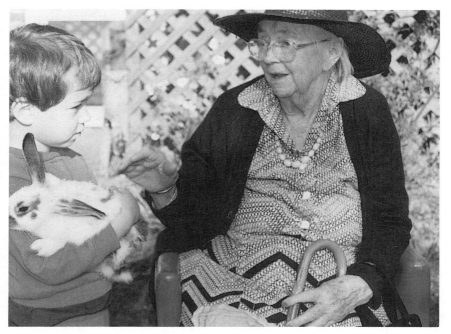

This little boy brings his pet rabbit with him to visit grandma.

Introducing constructive visiting

There are three main ways of introducing and developing constructive visiting:

- provide many social events and activities at which visitors are made to feel welcome
- develop a 'Visiting' leaflet which offers ideas on how to make visits more enjoyable
- develop an information video or leaflet which introduces the centre, the staff and the program to visitors — it should place particular emphasis on the important role the visitor has in the care of residents

Increased opportunity for normal contacts

Introduce social activities which encourage visitors to be involved in a normal way with their relative. Some ideas are:

Open days or fetes: These can include garden parties, brass bands, afternoon tea and fundraising. Visitors should be encouraged to help with their relative's mobility, meals and activities throughout the day.

Social events: Develop regular occasions for parties to which residents, staff and visitors are all invited. They create further chances for meaningful time with the resident and time to mix socially with staff. Some examples: weekend picnics and barbecues; concerts; evening socials on individual wards in the larger settings; costume balls (visitors can be invited to help make their relative's costume); formal dinner parties; outings; shopping trips and shows; calendar celebrations (see Chapter 5).

Touring and holidays: Weekend trips and holidays can be organised where visitors are invited to go along too (see Chapter 7).

Community involvement: Visitors can be involved with their relatives in community activities, senior citizens groups, social clubs, church groups, craft meetings and at local schools.

Happy hour: Beer, sherry, wine, lemonade, or a cup of tea can be provided at a time when visitors seem to gather naturally. Invite people to bring a plate. A good social atmosphere will develop spontaneously.

Involvement in regular activities: Visitors can be invited to assist, for example, with crafts, outings and small groups where one-to-one supervision is required. This will help them to feel they are contributing significantly to the life of their friend.

Volunteer service: Some visitors want to be regularly employed in assisting residents, both their own relatives and others. It is particularly ideal for those living alone after the spouse has been placed in extended care.

'Self-help' groups: Visitors should be encouraged to take the resident to local community groups, particularly those which the resident used to attend before moving into the centre.

Seasonal magazine: Visitors may like to help compile material for a homegrown magazine, or contribute to it. Include a calendar update of coming events which visitors are invited to attend.

Bulletins: Other special bulletins or letters and invitations can be distributed for the various special events which are occurring in the next month.

Visitors' leaflets

A 'Visiting' leaflet can be developed which suggests topics of conversation and ways to get around the problem of what to talk about. It could include a map of the centre, showing visiting areas, garden and courtyard areas to sit in, notice boards, shops and transport. It could also direct visitors to local attractions which are within walking distance of the centre.

The following sample of a visitors' handout was compiled by Kay Dannatt and may help you develop a handout for your own setting. A colourful pamphlet format would make the information more attractive (although a typed sheet is better than nothing!).

VISITING

Some information for visitors

Any staff member at . . . . could describe our residents' need for visitors; their constant comments and questions while waiting for visitors; their pleasure in describing family events and the proud discussion about various members of their family. It is the highlight of the day to receive a visitor. So, by trying to make your visits as meaningful and constructive as possible, you will contribute significantly to the quality of life of the resident. It is the most valued assistance you can offer to your loved one.

You may like to draw on this list from time to time; it is designed to make visits easier and more fulfilling for yourself and your relative. However, the best person to consult about preferred visiting activities and discussion ideas is the resident. Always find out how he or she is feeling, and what he or she would like to do today.

It can at times be difficult to make conversation. Although silence is golden, deadly silence can be most uncomfortable. Life can sometimes seem rather routine, which can limit conversation. Yet life at . . . . can be exciting and there is usually plenty to talk about. Later in this brochure is a list of 'conversation starters' to help get a discussion going.

Have you tried these ideas?

Walks: You are welcome to take your relative for a walk. If you need wheelchair assistance or even a nurse, this can be arranged. Nearby . . . . gardens are beautiful, or a visit to (a nearby attraction such as the beachfront or other place of interest) is always very pleasant.

Bus trips: We have access to a bus and you are welcome to join our drives and outings. See the activity coordinator and watch the weekly program sheet.

Join activities: You're welcome to join in the activity program throughout the week. Come to the Recreation Activities and feel free to join in bingo, crafts, parties, cooking, films, church or the garden club. Perhaps you could bring in some samples of craft that your relative or friend has done in the past, to show others.

This kind of participation will help you to familiarise yourself with your relative's daily activities, friends, and staff members. It will be easier to make conversation and ask questions. You can invite your relative or friend to describe what's been going on; remembering details, naming people, being oriented to various events, places and people.

Hobbies: Why not bring in your own activity or hobby? Bring your knitting or stamp collection and do it with your relative.

Games: Bring along a game, especially your relative's favourite. Choose draughts, chess, cards, crossword puzzles or jigsaws. Do it together. It is fun and mentally stimulating. We have games available for you to use as well.

Previous interests: Think about your friend's previous interests and hobbies. Look back over the years; with practice you can draw out his or her knowledge and create discussion. You will find you collect snippets of interest, making it a learning experience for you.

Letters: Write some letters with your relative, or greeting cards when appropriate. This encourages participation in family affairs and is a stimulating activity.

Newspapers: Try reading the newspaper or a favourite magazine together. Discuss the news and any interesting articles. This helps to keep your relative in touch with outside affairs. Include articles about events in the local community; discuss local identities and activities in which the resident may have been involved in the past.

Gifts: Use them as a conversation piece. For example, flowers can stimulate discussion about different seasonal flowers, where they are grown, the variety of colours, and so on.

Clothing: If one of you is wearing something different, comment on it; discuss its colour, texture, ask your friend's opinion of it.

Ask for advice: Ask for your relative's opinion on other subjects, such as a menu you are planning, recipes, changes in the home, gardening, places to go on outings, quality of shopping items.

Family events: If you have a special family event coming up such as a wedding, birthday or Christmas dinner, you may wish to involve your relative in some way. If you need some assistance or advice, please feel free to speak to the nursing or therapy staff, who will be happy to help.

Family photographs: Bring in family photographs, even the old family album. It makes for excellent conversation and can lead to a good laugh. Invite your relative to pick out some photographs to keep. Framing them may be a good activity for him or her to be involved in, and the photographs can then be hung in his or her room. Leave a small album of photographs for the resident to refer to at other times. Include family members, the family home, recent events of the centre.

Special events: We are always planning special events where the family may wish to be involved. You are most welcome to attend parties, barbecues, outings and concerts. This is an ideal time to spend with your relative, rather than just visiting.

Library: Your local library will have a supply of large pictorial books on nature, geography, travelling, and so on. The photographs provide interesting browsing and stimulate discussion.

Music   is a great 'get-together' tool. If you play an instrument or the grandchildren are learning, you are welcome to bring them in or to play the piano. Or bring tapes and records that you know are favourites. Anyone from the activity department can make the stereo system available to you. It is portable so you can use it anywhere in the building.

Some extra guidelines

Touch: If your relative is unable to converse with you, perhaps has poor eyesight, or is confused about where he or she is, it is sometimes soothing and pleasant just to sit and hold hands. This is reassuring for an anxious or blind person, as he or she can feel you are there. Using hand cream to massage the hands can also add pleasure to the visit. The staff may be able to supply appropriate cream for ageing skin, so feel free to ask.

Roster visits: It can be a good idea to make a family 'roster' for visiting. It's more beneficial for your relative to have several visitors spread over a time rather than all arriving at once, which can be a little overwhelming and tiring for an older person, especially around Christmas. If possible, involve the resident in planning the roster and make sure he or she knows who is coming and when.

Children: Encourage children to participate in communication with grandparents. They usually have endless projects and school work, especially things they have made, which can be taken to show and used as conversation starters.

Involve others: If conversation is difficult at times, invite other residents to join in. It helps to encourage social contacts among residents.

Community resources: Various community services offer assistance to those who live in small nursing homes and special accommodation houses where outings and activities may not be available. Inquire about the help which is available. For example, the council welfare officer may be able to arrange transport to the local senior citizens centre for lunch, or a trip home or to the bowling club.

Television: Avoid watching television while visiting (unless it's the resident's favourite program). Use the time instead to draw out news and gossip. If possible, turn off noisy radios or television sets — they are very distracting and residents have plenty of time to watch television. Visiting time is more precious.

Privacy: Don't sit in communal lounge rooms while visiting if it's possible to go elsewhere. Normal conversation is often difficult when others are listening. A stroll together somewhere is more private. You and your relative deserve privacy, and you'll find it much more relaxing. Of course, sometimes you may wish to join in a 'community lounge' visit, as it helps you and your relative to get to know the others and communicate more freely with them. You may both like to participate when something special is occurring at the centre.

Going out: Have you thought about taking your relative or friend out but decided it may be too difficult? Trained staff are willing to show you the easiest methods of handling disabled people. Getting in and out of cars, going up and down steps, getting on and off toilets, and so on, can all be barriers unless you know the simple method. Please inquire. There is also equipment available for loan or hire which may mean independence is possible and make the difference between going on an outing or remaining home-bound.

Chores: Are there some repetitive chores you do at home which your relative may like to help with? Forget your inhibitions and take along the handkerchiefs to be folded, silver to be polished, wool to be untangled or rolled, socks to be sorted, sewing box to be tidied, photographs to go in albums, carpentry tools to be cleaned, or even more difficult chores if they suit your relative's abilities and interests.

Reality orientation: Help your resident to remember where you are, what time it is, what the weather is like. Hang a calendar in his or her room to mark off special events: your next visit or birthdays. Don't correct your relative, just make it a part of the general conversation about the weather and seasons.

Jot down ideas: As you think of them, make a note of ideas you can use to chat about when you visit. This will make the visit far more constructive and help you to avoid repeating the same problems or stories.

Conversation starters

The occupational therapist can supply you with more conversation starters or subjects for discussion, if you need them.

- What's new at . . . . , new staff, new pictures, furniture?
- What's happening at . . . . , what did you do today?
- What's new out in the garden, new flower beds, trees with new leaves?
- What's on for dinner, how was lunch, what did you have?
- Discuss the weather, but extend to events that take place according to season, e.g. farming, gardens, food and vegetables, type of weather, summer events and holidays.
- The day of the week, what happens e.g. on Mondays (shopping?), at the weekend?

- What you saw on the way there, e.g. new facilities, traffic lights being put in, children out early from school.
- School news — holidays, fetes, what the children are doing.
- Report on family activities, however routine and simple.
- Who you have been visiting and what that person has been doing.
- Who you saw at the shops.
- What you have to buy on your next shopping trip.
- What shops have closed, new ones opened, or buildings been renovated.
- New products on the market; your resident will find it interesting to discuss modern products and new methods, e.g. for housework.
- Houses for sale in the area.
- Local festivals, e.g. arts festival, concerts, plays.
- If your friend is from another town, try to get that town's local newspaper. Talk about the town and where it is situated.
- Television programs, who's on, new shows. Ask your relative to describe favourite programs to you.
- Famous people gossip, e.g. the Royal Family, the Prime Minister, or new government, local members, or the Mayor.
- Plan a day out, e.g. It's a lovely sunny day today. Where would be a good place to go? What would you do?

(end of handout)

Making a video

A video can be made to show to relatives and friends of residents who have been recently placed. If the centre does not have the resources to make a video, a local school or college could be approached and students invited to make the video as part of their study projects.

The contents of the video could include an introduction to the centre, demonstrations of constructive visiting, details of who to approach for help, and the use of available equipment.

Introduction to the centre: This part of the video can feature staff members such as the manager and the medical director/geriatrician, who should tell relatives about the ageing process in simple terms, the importance of visitors, the multidisciplinary approach, and the residents' need for active participation in daily life. The director or deputy director of nursing should talk about the nursing aspects of placement, food and all other aspects of life on the ward. The video could also feature the welfare officer/social worker/liaison officer from the community, who can discuss the financial and practical details of a person entering the centre.

Demonstration: The second part of the video could deal with constructive visiting. Feature an occupational therapist or physiotherapist demonstrating to relatives or friends how to transfer residents in and out of a car or to negotiate steps. Aim to encourage viewers to take their relatives home for visits, or on outings, and demonstrate that plenty of help is available. The video could also show a nurse helping someone out of a car, and suggest that a nurse might be spared for a special outing or perhaps hired from an agency (if it can be afforded). The video should encourage the relatives to ask questions and express their needs.

Who to go to for help: Use the video to introduce staff members, as many visitors do not know who to approach to ask questions. For example, in a smaller nursing home, the Director of Nursing may answer all inquiries, yet many people may be afraid to approach her, or find it difficult to get in contact with her. In a larger hospital, who does one ask? The ever-changing sister in charge, a nurse, or the doctor? Relatives usually end up asking a neighbour for information which may sometimes be wrong. People need to know where and from whom they can get information and assistance.

Equipment: The video can demonstrate the use of equipment for people with disabilities and give information about its availability for outings and weekends away. If relatives are aware that they can borrow a wheelchair or commode, and know how to use it, they may be more easily encouraged to take their loved one home for a break or Christmas dinner.

Brochure

An alternative to the video could be a clearly printed brochure offering the same kind of information described so far. (Many hospitals do have leaflets available, but most tend to be filled with lots of other information.) The brochure could follow a question and answer style. It should pose the sorts of questions visitors usually want to ask, following each with a brief answer. For example: 'Who needs to know that I am taking a resident out for a while?' The answer may be the charge nurse or receptionist.

Throughout the video/brochure the main aims should be to encourage more visiting and clearly indicate a welcoming attitude from all staff. The information should be geared towards helping visitors, rather than confusing them with a lot of useless facts.

Conclusion

The importance of friends and relatives in the lives of people in aged care facilities cannot be underestimated. Normal contacts with people need to be maintained and encouraged to ensure real quality of life for residents. Many people from the community find the nursing home environment threatening. Some may be fearful of authority figures, or find that communal living makes visiting with privacy too difficult. Everything possible must be done to make the environment warm and encouraging. Visitors need to feel valued and, initially, they often need guidance to make their visits enjoyable for both themselves and their friend.

Reference

1. Schultz R. Effects of control and predictability on the physical and psychological well-being of the institutionalized aged. *Journal of Personality and Social Psychology*. 1976; 33(5).

Chapter 14
Older People with Dementia
with Adriana Tiziana, Eunice Barter
*and Madge Williams**

This chapter will discuss the special requirements of the confused older person, who has as much need for a lifestyle of quality as other more alert older people. Indeed, such a person is in greater need of assistance from others to maintain this quality. In many cases traditional activities may be too difficult, but this does not mean that people with confusion should be excluded from the activity program. As the centres described in this chapter suggest, quality of life should still be possible for the person with dementia.

All the principles and most of the activity ideas described in earlier chapters also apply to this group of people. Certainly, all the program ideas in this book have been applied to settings where a significant number of participants demonstrated various levels of dementia. Some activities will be too difficult for some people, and others may need to be presented in a different manner to enable people with dementia to participate successfully. This chapter provides guidelines to ensure that people with dementia can still participate actively in the life of the centre. (Refer also to Chapter 18 which describes how to adapt activities to match the abilities of the participants.)

A number of people who work in centres designed exclusively for people with dementia have been invited to describe their programs, and these examples can be used in the design of activity programs which have such participants in mind.

The chapter also includes a brief look at two approaches to the care of the confused: Reality Orientation and Validation Therapy. This overview

---

* Adriana Tiziana from the Alzheimer's Society contributed to the section on 'Approaches to the care of people with dementia.' Eunice Barter was director of the Gatehouse Day Centre and a lecturer at the Mayfield Centre. Madge Williams was a director of Sefton Lodge.

is designed to introduce the two methods to readers who are unfamiliar with them. It is not intended to give a blueprint for their application but to encourage further investigation, although there are some basic principles arising from both which can be applied immediately. The chapter concludes with a set of guidelines compiled from the centres and methods described.

Not all the answers to working with people with dementia will be found here. That task is beyond the scope of this book. The major aim of this chapter is to encourage further reading and training in this specialised field and, at the same time, to demonstrate that people with dementia can and should be encouraged to participate in activities designed to improve their quality of life.

The Lodge Program

Madge Williams, past director of Sefton Lodge, has provided this summary of the Lodge Program, which is run by the Community Services Division of the Uniting Church in Australia.

This account exemplifies an excellent approach to the care of the older person with dementia. It describes the ideal size and structure for any residential facility seeking to recreate for its residents a natural home environment with warmth and security. The program fosters an environment where the dignity and self-esteem of the residents is of paramount importance.

The Lodge Program was first established in May 1975 as a pilot program for individuals suffering from irreversible dementia. The motivation arose from the awareness of Uniting Church social workers that there was no adequate accommodation for individuals moderately affected by dementia — for the wanderers who could no longer be trusted to take care of themselves.

The proposed plan was to provide security, warmth and companionship in a family group, in a cottage-home environment in an ordinary street, and be part of the local community and be accepted by them. This would help to reduce residents' feelings of anxiety and hopelessness, and enhance their feelings of peace and dignity.[1]

A house was selected in Camberwell, Victoria, to cater for eight women. The success of the program was evidenced by the rapid appearance of new lodges, resulting in a total of four. More information on the Lodge Program can be found in the book, *Forgetting but not Forgotten.*[1]

Sefton Lodge in Hawthorn opened in August 1985 for the Uniting Church Lodge Program. It was specifically designed to meet the needs of these special people, using the knowledge gained from the experiences of earlier lodges.

Sefton Lodge

It is worth looking at the features of Sefton Lodge which make it so unique. Other centres may like to draw ideas from this overview to adapt to their own facilities in creating a more positive home environment for their residents.

Sefton Lodge was designed to house ten physically active people, moderately affected with dementia, offering nine permanent and one respite care bed. It has six single rooms and two double. Residents are given the choice of bringing with them their own furniture and treasured possessions. Familiar objects help them to feel more at home.

A communal toilet and shower is situated close to the bedrooms. A central toilet block enables staff to monitor the movement of the women more easily than with en-suites in each room. It makes it easier for the staff to shower the residents, and facilitates supervision to prevent blocked toilets and flooded showers. The communal shower room also serves as a meeting place with continuous comings and goings and bright conversation.

The outside of the house was designed to fit in with the older houses in the area. As the residents are wanderers, security is important, but they are not made to feel closed in. Security has been accomplished with a low picket fence and a normal gate, which the women can see over. The gate is kept locked but, once each person settles into the Lodge, it seems to be of no consequence. The low fence allows the residents to view the busy street, and the church opposite provides an interest with the comings and goings of the congregation.

The lounge room has cathedral ceilings and is large and spacious, with furnishings in pastel colours. There is a gas log fireplace and 'Lucky', the canary, sits in the bay window. The lounge, dining room and kitchen are all situated in the same area, as in any family home. The staff have a view of the lounge room as they work in the kitchen, but the residents are not made aware of being supervised.

The dining area has a large dining table, which can seat all the women. The residents help to set the table, prepare the vegetables, and wash the morning and afternoon tea dishes, so they are continuously in a domestic environment which they have been used to all their lives.

The dining area is also another good area for communication. The residents are served breakfast in their dressing gowns, and conversation is usually about yesterday's events, today's news, plans for the day, and the anticipation of special events. Visitors usually join us for morning and afternoon tea around the table, so that residents who have few visitors can share in the company. After lunch the women often join in a singalong. Large print song books without music allow them to concentrate on the words, while helping to maintain reading skills.

The activities room adjoins the dining room. It is also spacious and airy. There is a pianola which is used for singalongs or for listening to our resident pianist. Although suffering from dementia, she can still play the piano beautifully and is encouraged by staff to retain this skill.

The activities room has a good view of the garden and the clothes line. This is deliberately placed as the women enjoy hanging out the washing and, at first sign of rain, bringing it in again!

Washing is sorted and folded by the residents and they also help with light ironing. However, the staff need to keep an eye on these activities as it's not unusual to see one person pegging up the clothes and another taking them down. Although we have a clothes dryer, the women are not familiar with it, so damp clothes are draped around chairs to dry and there is a rush to remove unsightly bloomers when unexpected visitors arrive. We do use the room for craft as well.

Another feature in making the lodge a home is 'Blackie', a Labrador cross. After some discussion, the residents decided they would prefer a dog to a cat, so the Keysborough Animal Shelter was approached and the volunteer workers produced 'Blackie'. He came on a month's trial and when the residents were asked if we should keep him, the vote was unanimous in his favour. They love him and he them. He brings them much joy, and is absolutely spoilt by everyone.

Staff

Sefton Lodge was designed to be as much like a normal house as a large centre can be, but even the most beautiful house is not necessarily a home. In any home, it is the family living there that makes the house a home. It requires loving parents who have the time to play, talk and listen to their children. It is easy to supply shelter, food and clothing, yet people need more; they need love, understanding and acceptance. So the job of making a lodge a happy home falls on the staff.

The lodge staff are chosen because of their skills, their personality and their attitudes towards older people.

The job takes patience, a good sense of humour and a great deal of commitment to the ideals of the lodge program. It takes patience to refrain from screaming when something frustrating occurs over and over again; or from crying as you watch a beautiful woman behaving like a young child; or when you have been left with yet another mess to sort out. It takes commitment from the staff to allow the women into the kitchen, or to ask the residents to help them when it's much easier to do the job themselves.

It also takes patience and commitment to meet the lodge philosophy that the residents should be dressed in street clothes and look attractive at all times when, as soon as you turn your back, someone adds extra underwear on top, or uses a toothbrush to comb her hair. It takes persistence, and a touch of genius, to find hidden false teeth or spectacles.

Yet it is rewarding to see the women looking attractive and it helps to maintain their self-esteem. The hairdresser's visit is usually a highlight on Monday morning. Everyone enjoys the special care and attention they receive, and the chance to freshen their appearance for the week.

An individualised approach

An important benefit which results from the small size of Sefton Lodge is that the staff get to know each person as an individual. We also keep a social history of the person, with information about their past hobbies and personality. The program can then respond to the special characteristics of each person. We try to encourage everyone to maintain their skills, such as playing the piano or painting.

Too often older people in our society reach the stage where they feel they are useless and can no longer contribute to the community. We believe that by allowing the women to help with household chores, they feel needed and useful. This helps to maintain self-esteem and reduces feelings of helplessness. They clip stamps for the Uniting Church 'Sammy Stamp' appeal, and they also cut up old sheets and roll bandages for the leprosy missions. It is important that any activity the women do has a purpose. They often ask: 'Why are we making this, or doing that?' They need a satisfactory answer.

The program

As the program is structured around the residents, it is flexible. The daily program responds to the moods and preferences of the women on the day. We like to take them out for a morning walk to the park or the shops. We all go to the chemist to have prescriptions filled, to the post office or the paper shop. Each day the milk is picked up from the milk bar by the women. We could have it delivered, but collecting it is part of our reality program. We believe everything we do with the residents is reality orientation. To go to the bustling shopping centre, to push the button and cross with the green light, to be among busy shoppers and traffic is all very much a part of being in touch with the real world.

We take 'Blackie' up to the park for a run, stopping now and then to talk to children in strollers or to admire babies. Along the way we collect a few other dogs. It is interesting to see the number of people who stop to chat, or interrupt their gardening to say hello. Some of the residents collect flowers as they move around the streets and there are times when we have to pretend we don't see them. They press the flowers or arrange them in vases. We have one woman whose job it is to water and arrange the flowers; she does it well, so we encourage her to use this skill.

Regular outings occur in the Hawthorn community bus. We visited a tulip farm, where, much to the amusement of other visitors, our residents danced along to the music from the loudspeakers.

Music is very much a part of the lodge program. The residents do not always need the staff to lead them once a record is placed on the turntable, they will sing along or begin dancing to the music.

They attend church every Sunday morning. Members of the congregation pick them up and take them to the service. Most of them have always been church-goers and they continue to enjoy it.

Every second Tuesday they go to the local drop-in centre, where they play games such as bingo, with the help of the others who attend. The over-sixties club in Hawthorn picks them up on Sunday afternoons and takes them to their concert. Boys from Scotch College visit every Thursday and girls from the Methodist Ladies College also visit weekly. They give manicures and help with crafts. Student nurses from the Hawthorn Day Hospital visit twice a week.

We have a family Christmas carol service and annual centre birthday parties. Both are well attended by the residents' families. The mini-fete is another way to keep the family involved.

The garden offers a good source of activity. Seedlings are planted and weeds pulled. During the summer months, morning and afternoon tea is usually served outside. (It is important to have comfortable garden seats.)

Things we have learnt

- the limit for craft work is 30 minutes, because of the short concentration span
- music is important — our residents love to sing and they remember all the old songs
- they prefer to watch television only in the evenings — they like to see the news but find it difficult to follow picture stories, because of limited concentration
- they enjoy hearing funny poems, or listening to the Association for the Blind talking books
- they play games like I Spy or the Junior Trivia
- most of all they love fun — if laughter could cure, we would not keep our residents long
- some of the women need time out for themselves, although it's rare for any of them to stay in their rooms

The aim of the Lodge Program is to enable residents to attain maximum individual fulfilment within the limits of their disability, and to enjoy quality of life. We feel the success of the Lodge Program lies in its simplicity.

The Gatehouse Day Centre

The philosophy and approach behind the Sefton Lodge program was derived partly from its links with the Gatehouse Day Centre in Kew, Victoria. The program at the Gatehouse was established by Eunice Barter, RN, and is included here as an example of the kind of programs that can be developed for people with memory loss.

Aims of the centre

The Day Centre is attended by people with dementia who are being managed at home with their families. While providing carers with some respite, the centre also seeks to create a normal home environment which encourages residents to feel secure, respected and worthwhile. The program aims:

'to maintain or improve existing skills in independence in activities of daily living, to retrieve old skills such as gardening, meal preparation and socialising, to increase their awareness of who they are, and to improve their self-esteem and physical fitness.'

The basic premise of the program is that our clients should be treated just as the staff would expect to be treated themselves, that is, as valued adults. We seek to encourage and develop dignity and self-esteem in each individual.

The program

Ten participants attend each day, from 10am to 3pm. The program is run by 2 staff helped by 1 or 2 volunteers, and follows the normal pattern of the day. It begins with morning tea, a chat to help orient participants to their whereabouts and to each other, then warm-up activities. The focus then becomes preparing the lunchtime meal and clearing up afterwards. Lunch is followed by walks, rest for those who desire it, gardening, path sweeping and simple activities; or a staff member or volunteer may sit with one participant and look through their 'This is Your Life' book. Afternoon tea and a singalong complete the day.

'This is Your Life' book

Staff and relatives compile a 'This is Your Life' book for each participant, in which is recorded their family tree, their interests and hobbies, occupation, special skills, past achievements, war service, and so on, including photographs past and present. These books appear to provide participants with a great sense of identity and a past they clearly recognise. This simple idea is worth applying to any other aged care setting. It could become a project for school students to help compile these booklets as part of their literacy program.

Teamwork

Everyone operates as a team and staff work alongside participants. Many
forgotten skills can be re-activated simply because there is someone else
there to copy. Everything is achieved through example. It is far less threatening to observe and copy someone else who is peeling potatoes, for
example, than to have to wonder what on earth this odd piece of equipment is, and try to follow verbal instructions which can be confusing and
hard to remember. All activities are familiar and everyday, drawing on
special skills and past experiences wherever possible. For example, one
man who had been a photographer loves to look through photographs and
pictorial books.

The staff find that participants respond well to this approach. Since
most activities invite the participants to contribute significantly to the
running of the centre, a greater sense of self-worth and dignity is fostered.
As one woman was thanked for helping to clear the dishes, she exclaimed:
'Have I been helpful? I never seem to be of any use to anyone these days!'
Many families report that their relative is far more settled following a day
at the centre.

Guidelines

- participants are much happier to attend the centre if it is described as
  a club for people with a 'bit of forgetfulness' rather than a Day Centre
- everyone wears a name tag with their preferred first name to offer in-
  stant information to each other
- staff should work alongside participants, offering example rather than
  instruction

The Gatehouse Centre offers a very simple yet effective program which
can significantly improve the quality of life of its participants. It could
easily be applied to any other aged care setting, whether residential or
community-based. The warm, friendly, respectful environment at the
Gatehouse should be evident in every aged care facility, regardless of the
disabilities of the participants.

Approaches to the care of people with dementia

A brief overview of Reality Orientation and Validation Therapy is included here to offer food for thought when considering how to care for the
confused resident.

Both theories offer many valuable insights into this field of care, some
of which can be applied immediately to any setting. For example, the
Reality Orientation approach suggests giving clear verbal commentaries
on the various activities which are occurring around the individual.

Validation Therapy encourages a warm, accepting non-corrective manner when talking with the confused resident.

However, other aspects of these programs require a thorough understanding of the principles and careful application of the practices if they are to be successful. Consequently, further reading and, in some cases, training is advised before attempting the application of these methods. (See the end of this chapter for further reading, and Appendix B for details of training programs in aged care.)

Regardless of the approach that one takes, one of the essential factors which needs to be taken into consideration is personhood. Personhood is not easy to explain but Mary Buzzell in her paper *Personhood: The Vital Component in Gerontological Nursing* (1989)[2] explains it as:

'Different aspects of the person, particularly those unique characteristics, attributes and strengths which make each individual different from another and unique as a human being. Personhood is at the root of individual vulnerability. When it is honoured we feel comfortable. When it is not taken into account by others we feel depersonalised. Personhood consists further of our values, spirituality and our preferences welded together through years of living.

'Our experience shapes our personhood. To ignore a person's life experiences is not only to devalue the individual, but to render him vulnerable. The impact of experience can produce strengths and buffer us in the ups and downs of life. When these strengths are ignored by health professionals, the professionals take on too much of the person's total burden. This robs the individual not only of an opportunity for growth but also of the satisfaction of accomplishment.

'Above all, personhood is rooted in personal history and nurtured through years of living. It encompasses our personal likes and dislikes, needs and wants, beliefs and habits. It includes one's strengths, contributions and potential.

'By the time an individual reaches adulthood, he is in control of those parts of his environment which impinge upon his personhood. If the noise of television is bothersome, he can turn it off. If the individual is a night person, he can minimise morning stimulation. He is free to pursue his wishes and to have alternatives. He has gathered friends that reinforce his values. His history and roles are affirmed. He has carved a niche that ensures his comfort.

'In long term care, Personhood is often neglected or not acknowledged. At this time, in practice, it is rare for an organisation to give an individual enough control over his environment to ensure his comfort and protect his vulnerability. If the staff do not know he dislikes background noise, for example, he may well be placed in the noisiest section of the unit. His resultant behaviour may unjustly earn him the label of an angry cantankerous person. If he has been a loner all of his life, with a need for privacy, and this is unknown, a care plan may be initiated that includes attendance at groups. Small daily annoyances may make the difference between a good adjustment to long term care or a bad one.'

As health professionals caring for confused older people, we must ask ourselves 'how much do I know about this *person*? about his likes and dislikes? about the things that were important to him?' Aggressive and agitated behaviours have often been triggered because a person's 'person-hood' has been devalued. Mary Buzzell uses her Aunt Dorothy to illustrate the importance of personhood:

'My Aunt Dorothy is sitting with her two sisters Al and Miriam by her side. She was a quiet, gentle person who was very comfortable being alone. She walked four miles a day and enjoyed doing crossword puzzles by the hour. When acute glaucoma caused her to lose her vision, she asked me one day for a favour, a rare event. She knew her time of living alone was nearing an end and that she would soon move to a long term care facility. Aunt Dorothy asked me to speak on her behalf, to tell staff that she enjoyed her aloneness, lest it be interpreted as aloofness or loneliness. She wanted me to convey, for her, that she was not a group person, not a joiner. Her personhood, like that of other adults was rooted in her life history and yet it is precisely one's life history that is often amputated on admission to our care.'

It is probably a good time to ask ourselves the same questions. What is important to me? What do I really enjoy? (e.g. sleeping in, strong black coffee, classical music). How would I feel if these things were taken away from me or I was subjected to those things which I really dislike? (e.g. woken up at 7am with a weak white tea!)

To return to Reality Orientation and Validation Therapy, as previously stated successful application of these principles requires thorough understanding, and the acknowledgement of each person with dementia as a person who has good and bad days. Practices which previously worked may not continue to work as the disease progresses.

Reality Orientation

Reality Orientation is an approach which seeks consistently to orient the confused person to the 'here and now'. Staff are trained to introduce the time of day and immediate surroundings into their everyday conversations with residents, in order to remind them who and where they are. It proposes to disrupt cognitive decline by stimulating the confused individual with repetitive activities on an individual or group level. Reality orientation takes three main forms:

The 24 hour approach

This is sometimes also referred to as continuous reality orientation. Name, date, time and other facts or orientation are reinforced and ideally, it is used by every person interacting with the confused person.

The 24-hour approach seeks to encourage staff to relate well and communicate clearly with residents, respecting their dignity and self-esteem. This is achieved by providing them with accurate information about all the events occurring to them and around them. Residents are not corrected or reminded of details, but simply kept up-to-date. Normal conversation includes such statements as: 'Hi, Mary, it's Anne here. I've come to help you get up this morning.' The staff member may discuss details of getting up and include information about the day's activities, which help to identify its place in the week.

Reality orientation groups

This is a more formal approach. It can include discussing the date, the weather and each other's names. It is followed by discussion of the past and present to encourage socialisation and learning. Participants can also join in other activities suited to their abilities.

If not handled carefully, this approach can begin to resemble that of a classroom, which is somewhat demeaning for its participants and outside 'normal' experiences for older people.

It is also very important to diagnose correctly and group people appropriately, according to their levels of confusion. There is a story of a 95-year-old resident who was once included by a keen therapist in a reality orientation group. The woman later expressed concern to the Director of Nursing that one so young should not know which day of the week it was!

Prescribed attitudes approach

Here staff determine a consistent approach which will be used by all staff with a specific resident. For example, kind firmness, active friendliness, or a matter-of-fact approach. The approach is chosen according to the person's personality and needs. (Note that a different approach may be needed in different situations, so it can be difficult to apply.) To some, this approach may seem too manipulative. In addition, no studies seem to have been carried out to test its value.[3]

One or all of these approaches can be used. However, the second and third forms of reality orientation do not work well without the first one. Various control studies have demonstrated some significant improvement in, and maintenance of, orientation, concentration, memory and conversational skills, where the 24-hour and group methods have been applied. However, they have also found that deterioration occurs if the program is discontinued.[3] It is important to note that programs should not be started if they cannot be maintained over time.

Staff training is necessary to ensure that the program is applied correctly, consistently and with the support of everyone. Without careful training the approach can be misused. It should also be noted that reality orientation should not be applied in a vacuum but as part of a total program which includes socialisation and recreational programs.

Validation therapy

Validation looks at old age in terms of the total life cycle of an individual and the differing goals which each individual seeks to achieve at each stage. It works on the premise that there is a reason behind all behaviour. Old age is a time for life review, for tying up loose ends in the preparation for death. Disorientation is considered to be a way of dealing with disordered thinking, replacing it with feelings.

Validation is a process where the individual can return to times in her life when she felt valued, useful and loved. It de-emphasises the relevance of orientation facts to the older person. The approach recommends that carers recognise and respond to the person's fantasy, acknowledging its reality and importance to that person. Together with warmth, caring and empathy, this encourages the person to respond to the carer and to interact more readily with others. It may slow deterioration. Some may even choose to return to reality.

Although much dementia is caused by physical disorders which are irreversible, so that real improvement cannot be observed, there is much that makes sense about the validation approach. A warm, respectful approach which validates and recognises the worth of the person is known to reduce agitation and the need for medication, and to improve the quality of life of the individual. Many workers may already apply some of this approach without realising that a method exists within which to place it.

Naomi Feil's books *Validation. The Feil Method*[4] and *The Validation Breakthrough*[5] are useful references. Other more recent articles on this method are available through most paramedical libraries.

One study[6] attempted to determine if either reality orientation or validation therapy had any effect on cognitive status, functional status or level of depression. Although this study has its own limitations, the following points are interesting to note:

- reality orientation failed to have an effect on mental status, activities of daily living (ADL) or life satisfaction (as identified in other studies)
- results of validation therapy are consistent with the only published study on validation therapy, which found no effect on mental status or morale

One of the challenges in caring for people with dementia is to try various methods and determine what works for the individual rather than looking for 'cure-alls' or a solution to the problem. The reality of the situation is that caring for people with dementia is challenging and there are no easy answers!

The value of musical quizzes

Music is a great source of pleasure and stimulation for people with confusion. Betty Stinson is an occupational therapist, who worked with confused people at Overton Nursing Home in Kew. She found that music became a very significant part of her program. Background music can be confusing to people with dementia, particularly those with an additional hearing loss, but music as an activity can bring much pleasure and revive old memories and abilities.

Betty Stinson has devised a number of musical quizzes which have been particularly successful. These quizzes offer a rare opportunity for the confused person to exhibit and experience considerable skill in an activity. Care must be taken to select songs from the era which matches the experiences of the group members. (See also Chapter 8 on music and Appendix F for song titles from different eras.)

Song quizzes

- sing the first line of a song and ask the group to finish it
- follow the themes of the year — ask the group to think of songs from a specific country or event, e.g. Australiana, Irish songs, love songs for St Valentine's day, and so on (see Chapter 5)
- ask the group to think of songs which mention colours, animals, flowers, birds, cities of the world, or a certain first name
- remember and sing songs from the first and second world wars

In each case, sing the songs together. Refer to Appendix F for song titles for each of these themes.

Word quizzes

Some associative word games can also stimulate automatic memory recall, and they offer a chance for participants to succeed in an activity. The following ideas have proved useful. Word association games can be found in many word game books.

- beginnings of proverbs (a stitch in time . . . .) or word associations (a fork and . . . .)
- leading ladies; guess their partners
- give the surname of famous personalities from the past and ask the group for the first name

Use all these quizzes to encourage reminiscing. Discuss and share the memories they trigger. A volunteer, who is from a similar era and the same local area as the participants, may like to research material to devise age and experience related quizzes.

Working with people with dementia

The following guidelines summarise the important principles and practices to consider when working with the person with dementia.

- Respect the dignity of each individual. Give people the same respect and care that you expect from others.
- Recognise the histories of people and the contributions they have made in the past. However, it is important to also recognise that history can lead a person to not want to participate or to respond negatively to a particular activity.
- Recognise that a person who is confused is subject to many fears, which can enhance behavioural disorders. A calm, secure, supportive environment allays fear and can significantly reduce distressed and abnormal behaviour. It also seems to reduce the need for drug therapy and its incumbent inadequacies.
- Use preferred names of both participants and staff.
- Avoid uniforms and authority structures. These can create fear and unnatural relationships between participants and staff. Everyday clothes help to foster a more homelike environment and place everyone on the same level, encouraging normal friendships to develop.
- Work towards developing warm lasting friendships.
- Use gentle touch to guide movements and encourage warm interaction. (But use touch with caution.)
- Speak clearly; explain your actions simply, one task at a time.
- Use familiar activities, both everyday activities and those which draw on the past experiences of each individual.
- Make sure activities are achievable and appropriate, and do not cause frustration.
- Use activities which stimulate a variety of senses — visual, taste, smells, textures.
- Draw on automatic responses to assist achievement, as in word games. Use familiar tasks from the past.
- Do everything together; provide examples rather than instruction.
- Limit activities to short periods of time to suit reduced concentration spans.
- Work in a distraction-free environment; specifically, no background television or radio.
- Make talking and listening the main focus of all activities. Offer cues to assist the person's talking and actions.
- Music contributes significantly to the atmosphere and to a sense of well-being and pleasure. However, it can inhibit interaction between people

with hearing difficulties when used simply as background music. Make the music the centre of the activity.
- Go on weekly outings to places which are known to be meaningful to individual residents.
- Be aware of the complicating factors of depression. Ensure accurate diagnosis and psychiatric intervention where necessary. The depressed person needs to be listened to, reassured and comforted. Again, the key role of all staff in helping the depressed person is talking and listening. A willingness to get involved in the life of that person is essential.

Alzheimer's Society of Victoria (Previously known as ADARDS)

This is a society of support groups for carers of people with dementia. Its aims are:

- to develop support groups within the community to give families and other carers of affected persons an opportunity to assist and encourage one another and to share and discover information about Alzheimer's disease and other related disorders
- to educate and inform the public, and medical and helping professions
- to advise government authorities on the needs of the affected persons and their families
- to promote research and seek to improve services for people with Alzheimer's disease and related disorders

See Appendix A for contact details.

Conclusion

This chapter is by no means comprehensive, and further reading and training are recommended. As a result of the programs illustrated here, it is hoped that people with confusion will not be excluded from activities. Their need for quality of life is as great as that of any other older person.

References

1. Marshall E, Eaton D. *Forgetting but not Forgotten. Residential Care for Mentally Frail Elderly People.* Division of Community Services: Uniting Church in Australia, 1984. A very useful text for those designing centres for people with dementia.
2. Buzzell M. *Personhood: The Vital Component in Gerontological Nursing.* Conference Paper, Sixth Annual Nursing Clinical Day, Bay Crest Centre for Geriatric Care, Toronto. 1989.
3. Holden UP, Wood RT. *Reality Orientation: Psychological Approaches to the Confused Elderly.* Edinburgh: Churchill Livingstone, 1982. A useful book for those

interested in this approach; a section headed '101 Ideas for Formal Reality Orientation Sessions' has some good ideas for discussion and reminiscing groups.

4. Feil N. *Validation. The Feil Method. How to Help Disoriented Old People*. Edward Feil Production, 4614 Prospect Ave, Cleveland, Ohio 44103.
5. Feil N. *The Validation Breakthrough*. Sydney: MacLennan and Petty. 1993. Originally published by Health Professions Press, Baltimore.
6. Scanland S.G. & Enershaw L.E. Reality Orientation and Validation Therapy. *Journal of Gerontological Nursing*. 1993; 19(6).

Further reading

Butler RN, Lewis MI. *Aging and Mental Health: Positive Psychological and Biomedical Approaches*. CV Mosby, 1982.

Shaw MW, ed. *The Challenge of Ageing*. Melbourne: Churchill Livingstone, 1983.

Chapter 15

The Larger Institution

with contributions from the late Mary Jones and amendments by Tania Agnew*

The information in this chapter is intended to dispel those comments often heard from staff of large geriatric institutions: 'But your centre is smaller and doesn't have the problems we have.' Although there are more hurdles and barriers to overcome, it is not impossible to introduce quality of life programs into these larger settings.

Some hierarchical and bureaucratic obstacles do exist in many larger settings. Unions are often averse to the use of volunteers, and the red tape involved in organising anything can become neverending. However, the residents of large institutions have perhaps a far greater need for these programs in order to work against the inevitable institutionalisation created by sheer size.

Communication can be the greatest obstacle

Many nurses and other staff who care directly for residents in large settings feel that the management structure is just too oppressive to begin introducing worthwhile programs. However, I have found that management is usually as committed to the quality of life of its residents as are other staff. (It needs to be remembered that very large centres are government-funded and not geared solely to profiteering.) The greatest barrier seems to be one of communication. One group of staff does not know how to convey its concerns in such a way that other groups will hear and respond positively. Certainly, each group will feel it knows a better way of achieving the goal of improved quality of life, and often the ways will differ greatly. However, a good starting point is to recognise that management and 'hands-on' carers do share this same goal.

Most often carers want as much freedom as possible to do their job well; management is usually concerned with maintaining tight controls to

---

* Tania Agnew is Recreation Manager at The Queen Elizabeth Centre, Ballarat, Victoria.

ensure that residents' rights and the centre's interests are not abused. In this case, some important communication structures need to be established to build trust and to help each group understand the others' reasons for their preferred methods of operation. (Some suggestions for this process will be described later.)

In addition, the larger setting requires a carefully designed coordinating structure to ensure that every resident has access to the activities provided. The sheer size and number of people to be catered for can itself be daunting. There will never be enough staff to go round. However, if the activity department seeks to be a resource service for other staff and volunteers rather than trying to provide all the activities itself, the task of giving everyone the chance to participate in activities does not seem quite so impossible.

Putting it into practice

Despite these hurdles, there are many larger institutions which do recognise the need for activity programs that work towards improving the quality of life of residents. They are finding that it is worth the effort to whittle away at the obstacles, in the interests of their residents' well-being.

I am certain that all the activity ideas and programs described in this book can be applied to the larger setting, and the best way to prove this is to give an example. To do this, we will take a look at the approach used by The Queen Elizabeth Centre, Ballarat, Victoria, to introduce activities and quality of life programs to its residents.

No place is perfect. Yet the model it provides for the introduction and coordination of activity programs in a large facility is a good one. Activity is becoming more and more a natural part of the life of the residents there.

Size is a substantial barrier to the creation of a homelike environment for residents. The Queen Elizabeth Centre, Ballarat, recognises that large institutions are not ideal for caring for older people, and is gradually introducing smaller centres throughout the region, which will one day take over the role of the large institution. Many other large geriatric centres throughout Australia are also moving in this direction. However, the Queen Elizabeth Centre also recognises the need to provide a decent quality of life for the residents who do have to cope with the present reality of large-scale, institutional living. The residents on the long-term wards should not be forgotten.

The late Mary Jones, coordinator of activities at The Queen Elizabeth Centre, Ballarat, described the centre and the methods they are using to break down the barriers.

This section begins with a description of The Queen Elizabeth Centre, Ballarat, to indicate clearly the size of the centre and the nature of its services. This is followed by a description of the organisational structure of the socialisation and activity program, which encourages all wards in this large setting to participate. It provides a useful model of a structure which can be applied to most other centres.

The Queen Elizabeth Centre, Ballarat

The Queen Elizabeth Centre, Ballarat, is located in Ballarat and, together with other organisations, services the health and welfare of aged and disabled people in the Greater Ballarat district and the Central Highlands region. Programs of assessment, rehabilitation, continuing care, education and research, undertaken within the centre and the community, are basic elements of the service network.

Services provided by the Queen Elizabeth Centre, Ballarat

Rehabilitation or restorative care

This service provides opportunities for disabled people to develop the ability to function at their maximum level of independence, and to return home, with support services if necessary. The service offers comprehensive rehabilitation, home adaptation and skills retraining to assist the person in this process. This is undertaken through the Rehabilitation and Assessment wards which have 45 beds, and a day hospital.

Regional services

The Queen Elizabeth Centre, Ballarat, offers advice and assistance to other smaller hospitals in the wider region. This is achieved through regular visits by a consultant geriatrician, welfare nurse and paramedical staff from the Centre. It is also achieved through the provision of educational programs to the staff of these centres.

Domiciliary services

A wide range of domiciliary services is provided by the centre, complementing programs provided by various local government and other agencies. These include:

- Home assessments and monitoring of individual client care.
- Linen service — bed linen, towels and draw sheets.
- Hot delivered meals for weekend and public holidays to supplement the Meals-On-Wheels service.
- Personal alarm call service: a radio transmitter, worn by the user, can be used to transmit a signal to the QEC,B in an emergency. Assistance is then summoned. A daily monitoring service is also provided.
- Accommodation — 66 flats are available for independent living.
- Emergency in home respite — provides the carer with a paid assistant until more permanent arrangements can be made.

- Outings/holidays — people receiving these services have the opportunity to take part in programs organised by the Centre.
- The Program of Aids for Disabled Persons (PADP) is a government funded program. The QEC,B acts as an issuing centre for the local region. It provides a variety of aids and equipment to help keep people in their own home.

Day centre care

Day centres are available which clients can attend each week. The program provides clients with:

- a chance to get out of the house
- social activation and companionship
- bathing, if required
- a hot midday meal
- transport to and from the day centre
- access to QEC,B services, if required
- continued monitoring of the general health and level of independence of clients

The Queen Elizabeth Centre, Ballarat operates four day centres, one of which is dementia specific. This day centre provides programs which focus on the individual needs of people, including weekend and overnight care.

Hostel care

Frail but reasonably independent people who need some assistance to cope with daily living activities and who have been assessed as requiring this level of care can be admitted to a hostel.

Six off-site hostels are situated north, south and west of the main centre.

Nursing home care

Extensive care is provided for people who have physical or mental disabilities which create dependency in one or more areas of functional activity.

Average age at admission is 79 years. The wheelchair population is about 65%.

The 402 beds are divided into 46–60 bed units. Each ward is therefore quite large in itself.

Non-clinical support services

The departments of the Corporate Services Division, such as Finance, Catering, Engineering, Ground & Gardens, Supply, Library, Environmental Services, Linen and Security, all play vital roles in the life of the centre. In addition to providing their specific functions, the staff from each department are encouraged to develop friendships with residents and, where possible, invite residents to participate in their activities. The Ground and Gardens Department has a particular commitment to making the gardens accessible to residents. Residents are invited to care for various raised garden areas and are welcome to pick flowers wherever they wish. The staff from the Environmental Services Department is in a particularly good position to get to know individual residents and form lasting friendships with them.

Socialisation Program

The socialisation program at The Queen Elizabeth Centre, which is designed for the long-term care residents, is perhaps the most distinctive feature of this large centre. Socialisation activities and recreation have a prominent place in the daily life of the centre.

To be successful, this program depends on the interaction of paramedical staff with staff from other areas. Recreation staff and assistants provide the base for many of the activities. Nurses are encouraged to participate fully in activities and to initiate many themselves. (This is discussed later.) The Occupational Therapy and Physiotherapy Departments offer advice and direction where necessary. Because the therapy departments have few staff hours available to give to the long-term sections, they have taken on a consultancy role.

Socialisation committee

A number of years ago senior management recognised the need to review its socialisation program and created a structure which would better coordinate the provision of activities and provide a clearer structure for communication between themselves and the various departments. It collected together representatives from nursing, activity, recreation and paramedical staff to form a committee whose functions were:

- to develop measurable objectives for socialisation
- to assess and monitor staff and volunteer resources
- to develop protocols for planning activities
- to oversee planning of seasonal activities
- to liaise between nursing, paramedical, volunteer sections and management
- to promote education and leadership skills
- to assess the needs of residents and dependency levels

The committee was instrumental in developing better lines of communication between various departments. It created clearer and simpler requisition processes for the organisation of various events, and established ongoing inservice training seminars for nurses, to encourage their greater participation in the socialisation process. Once it achieved its goals the committee was no longer needed and the recreation department assumed responsibility for the ongoing coordination of the socialisation program.

Objectives

The objectives for the provision of the socialisation program are simple, yet very important:

- to supply a large variety of quality of life programs to cater for the needs and wishes of the long-term care residents in the nursing home
- to be sensitive to the needs of the frail older and disabled residents, especially their need to be considered as individuals with a right to respect and dignity
- to develop and implement programs designed to maintain the highest physical, mental and social levels for residents

These objectives aim to reach each individual resident, offering everyone the chance to benefit from the stimulation programs. In addition, the aim is to provide a program which is varied, ongoing and occurs regularly.

Features of the Program

Socialisation assessment occurs routinely for each new person admitted to the centre. This helps to ensure that the program responds to the interests and needs of the residents.

Another important feature of the socialisation program is the role which the Recreation Department plays in resourcing the rest of the centre with ideas and materials for activities. This includes the provision of a resource book for each of the wards.

Each of these features is described more fully below.

Socialisation Assessment

A socialisation assessment is undertaken as part of the admission process for each resident. This ensures that staff are familiar with the interests of each person on their ward, and can encourage people to participate in activities which match their interests. The assessment is updated regularly to make sure that it reflects the current status of the resident. The results of all the assessments can also be compiled to survey which activities are generally most popular; this will assist in the selection of activities for program planning.

The form used is reproduced in Chapter 17.

Ward resource folder

A significant feature of the program at the QEC,B is the resource folder, compiled by the Recreation Department, to assist all staff in the planning and implementation of activities. A copy of the resource folder is available on each ward. This is an ongoing project with new ideas and resources being added as they are discovered and tested.

This is a particularly important method of disseminating information throughout a large institution. The Recreation Department then becomes the hub of a larger centre which is actively participating in a variety of activities at many different times during the day.

As a result far more people are able to take part in activities than if the activities room alone was the place in which to do activities. It also ensures that activities are not restricted to the working hours of the activity staff. It is an ideal model for larger extended care centres.

The resource folder contains the following information:

- lists of all equipment and games which can be borrowed from the Hook Centre with instructions on how to borrow them
- guidelines for conducting various activities such as outings, dinner parties and luncheons
- sample crosswords, word games, quizzes, plus advice about other games which are available for borrowing
- games and instructions for playing them, especially low-key games for very frail and wheelchair residents
- other ideas for spontaneous and planned activities on ward

To assist in this process of resourcing the centre, a monthly calendar is drawn up by the recreation staff. This calendar includes the Hook Centre schedule, on-ward activities, activities in other venues, outings and special events. The program is then circulated to all wards and participating staff. A noticeboard in the front foyer also displays daily happenings for residents and visitors entering the centre.

Activities

Any of the activities outlined in this book can be applied to the larger setting and the model of staff communication and participation described here will assist greatly in their application to such settings. The following description of available venues and their usage gives an indication of the scope of activities which can occur in the larger setting. Most large institutions will have areas which could be used for similar purposes.

Program venues

The F G Hook Centre is a ground floor, former day centre area that has been refurbished to function as an off-ward day centre area for long-term residents. A wide variety of individual and group activities is undertaken here each day:

- craft activities for residents who are able to work with minimal assistance and instruction — several 'work' almost full time at their hobby
- group activities in craft, woodwork and gardening are offered on a short sessional basis, once or twice weekly for the more dependent residents
- social groups such as bingo, cards, discussion groups and classical music
- individual quiet reading, watching television and playing music of their own choice
- special groups on a sessional basis such as pottery, moulded ceramics and painting
- special 'one-off' activities — Pancake Day, home-cooked lunches, or demonstrations
- armchair travel, monthly
- the F G Hook Centre Hall is also used regularly for community singing, school concerts and indoor bowls

The F G Hook Centre also acts as a resource centre for staff and volunteers — they can borrow equipment, resource materials and obtain advice. Other venues include:

- Lederman Hall (large hall with theatre stage), provides the venue for major functions involving very large groups of residents, such as Christmas, Easter and other special events
- on the wards there are sunrooms and lounges where daily individual and small group activities can occur
- outdoors — extensive gardens provide opportunities for walks, privacy, time with visitors and gardening (including many raised garden beds which residents can tend); there is also a barbecue area for picnics

Staff

Eight recreation members and five therapy nurses are employed to lead and organise socialisation programs in the nursing home for both individuals and groups. These staff also offer advice and direction to nurses wishing to organise activities at ward level.

Therapy nurses are now positioned on most units, and their role is to develop and manage the ongoing socialisation program appropriate to the needs and interests of the residents in the unit.

The QEC,B provides nurses with seminars on activities, encouraging them to make every activity, whether routine personal care or recreation, a pleasurable time for residents, for example, grooming can become a shared activity. Taking care to use separate, disposable applicators, makeup or a manicure could be done together; newspapers read together and articles swapped; a quick batch of scones whipped up; or a walk to the local park organised. Part of the education process includes helping nurses to look carefully at their work tasks to ensure that they do not use precious time which could be spent chatting to residents doing unnecessary tidying or documentation.

As a result, one ward at the centre reported that, since they have had a planned program of at least one social activity each day, the residents are much happier and brighter, and less dependent on staff. Those staff who participate in these activities find they also enjoy their work far more.

Volunteers

Interested and caring people have been recruited to participate and supplement the activities organised by staff. Areas of participation range from individual visiting to participating in larger group activities such as community singing and outings. The coordinator of volunteers is responsible for the recruitment, selection, orientation and education of volunteers. (For further information on volunteers, see Chapter 10.)

Community experience program

Students from many secondary schools attend each week to gain service experience, to learn about the care of frail older people and to develop friendships. Although this component requires a good deal of staff support, the benefits are immeasurable. The coordinator of volunteers organises this program, while activity and nursing staff offer ongoing supervision and direction (see Chapter 11).

Improving communication in the larger setting

At a management level, structures should be in place to enable staff representatives from all departments to make direct communication with senior management. This could be achieved by establishing a regular meeting between management and staff representatives. Alternatively, one or two staff representatives could be elected to attend relevant management meetings or sub-committee meetings. Likewise, it may be appropriate for some senior staff to be invited to attend the staff meetings of other departments from time to time.

The managers of the centre must work hard to involve both staff and residents in decisions which affect the lives of the residents. Management must also make it clear to everyone that they support the active involvement of staff members in the lives of the residents. People who enjoy their work are far more likely to work efficiently and, more importantly, offer a high standard of care to residents.

Inservice education is an appropriate forum for discussing with other staff the importance of activity programs which aim to improve quality of life. In addition, activity staff need to be prepared to speak at meetings of other staff groups, where appropriate, to encourage participation.

Informal communication has a part to play. Wherever possible, those who are involved in activity provision should encourage other staff to participate in the activities. A positive, involving approach which invites other people's ideas and contributions will work best in developing the enthusiasm of other staff.

Conclusion

The information in this chapter is supplied to encourage workers in the larger settings to apply the principles and practices described throughout the book. It recognises the special problems that larger settings face, and offers a structural base to make the application of these programs possible. Use the guidelines in Chapters 1 and 2 to underpin the activity program.

OCCUPATIONAL THERAPY

Chapter 16

The Occupational Therapist as Consultant

The following four chapters look briefy at the occupational therapist's role in extended care facilities and demonstrate the value of the services she can offer to this field.

Specialist skills

The services an occupational therapist can bring to an aged care centre are extensive — her expertise in design and access, adaptation of aids for independence, activities of daily living, disability handling, functional assessment and treatment for both physical and psychological conditions, activity analysis, program design and community resource skills make her a very useful person to know!

The occupational therapist has a significant role to play in the long-term care setting. She can assist in the assessment of people before they enter the home to ensure appropriate placement, and help the person to remain as independent as possible in the various activities of daily living. She can help to plan and adapt activities which the older person can participate in, despite disabilities. She can also observe potential areas where residents may be able to regain improved physical and/or mental functions, developing activities with that person to assist in the return or maintenance of these functions. And she brings with her a knowledge of a wide range of activities from which to develop a varied program.

These are all important services which should be accessible to every older person in residential care, to make sure that their quality of life is maintained at an optimum level.

Who should be the activity coordinator?

In the past the occupational therapist has usually filled the dual role of activity coordinator and therapist. This is quite an appropriate one; the occupational therapist's knowledge of activity and its adaptation, and her skills in fostering independence and improved quality of life for people, go well together.

However, as occupational therapists are in short supply, few can be found to fill the nursing home positions. Fortunately, other professional groups concerned with activity and recreation are now moving into the field of aged care. Recreation officers and diversional therapists are among those who can aptly fill the role of activity coordinator in the described settings. However, the other specialist skills offered by the occupational therapists are still needed in the aged care setting.

A new model is needed to respond to the changing availability of the various professional groups. The role of the physiotherapist is also changing. Few are available to give direct ongoing service to residents in long-term care, yet many residents require maintenance physiotherapy. Who is going to provide this necessary service?

Apart from the limited supply of these professional groups, the changing nature of aged care facilities will affect the availability of funding for these services. As centres become smaller and, therefore, more homelike, the funding made available for therapists is severely reduced. An alternative model is needed, one that is far more efficient.

The occupational therapist as consultant

As few occupational therapists are available to fill the nursing home positions, it seems that most centres make do without them at present. They rely, instead, on untrained activity workers to organise activities. A more appropriate alternative is to employ someone with recreation skills. This person will have the skills necessary to respond to the needs and interests of residents, and the ability to plan and implement many creative programs. A consultant occupational therapist can then contribute to the team of carers, visiting to offer advice and assistance in the areas of disability handling, activity adaptation, activities of daily living and program design.

The occupational therapist could be employed at the regional level, visiting various centres as required. Or a centre could employ her for an agreed number of hours to fulfil this role. Similarly, the physiotherapist could also assume a consultant role, directing an Allied Health Assistant, for example, to provide various maintenance programs for the residents.

Relevant experience

It is important, however, for the consultant occupational therapist to gain relevant experience in aged care, in order to understand the special needs of older adults. This can be gained by working in geriatric rehabilitation, day hospitals or community health centres. But I would suggest that some experience working in a centre and actually planning programs for people in residential care is particularly desirable. It may be difficult to encourage staff to participate, and to help restructure a program, if one cannot draw on one's own experience and verify that the suggested programs can be done!

The occupational therapist's role

The occupational therapist can then be employed to advise and support the activity coordinator. She can help to adapt activities and equipment to enable those with disabilities to participate more fully in the program and other activities of daily living (see Chapter 18). She can assist in assessment and program planning for each individual (see Chapter 17). The centre may call on her skills to redesign some of the facilities to encourage better access. She may also bring to the setting a wide range of resource material and take part in the inservice training program at the centre.

Activities of daily living

As described in Chapter 1, autonomy and independence can add significantly to a person's sense of well-being. However, it is important for the resident herself to determine the level of independence that she wants to exercise. Everyone should be encouraged to maintain the abilities they have, within reason. If a person's effort to get dressed is so great that she is too tired to enjoy the rest of the day, her right to request assistance should be respected. Another person may feel the effort is worth it, to maintain that sense of self-control.

The occupational therapist can play an important part here, by helping the resident to discover the level at which she would like to be independent and offering adaptations where necessary. The decision can then be recorded in the nursing notes, to make other staff aware of each person's preferences. Changes can be observed by all relevant staff over time.

It is particularly important to offer every opportunity for each individual to maintain independence at mealtimes, as this is a crucial area in maintaining personal control. In order to gain pleasure from food, one needs to determine which foods to eat when, at what speed, and in what quantity. It is difficult for even the most sensitive helper to discern and respond to these preferences. The occupational therapist can offer some very simple advice about aids and positioning which will help most people to maintain some degree of independence and control over their meals.

The home should offer every opportunity for the resident to choose to be involved in as many personal daily activities as would someone in their own home. The employment of a consultant occupational therapist will make sure this happens.

Team approach

The model proposed here needs to maintain a close team approach to service provision. Although they operate as consultants, the occupational therapist and physiotherapist will need to work closely with the other staff who have daily contact with residents. Regular meetings will be needed to exchange notes and to advise each other of the changing status of individual residents. The nurse and other staff who come into daily contact with residents will always remain the 'experts' because of their knowledge of each resident and his or her needs.

Conclusion

The consultancy role needs to be considered carefully by both occupational therapists and administrators of aged care facilities. It is also an issue which needs to be addressed by government departments as they consider the funding requirements for aged care facilities. This model needs to be developed further, to work towards better standards of care for all residents in all such centres in the future.

Chapter 17
Observational Assessment

Consider, for a moment, the circumstances of a person who has just arrived to be admitted to a nursing home. Can anyone comprehend the pain which this person must be going through as she faces the reality of her losses as a result of this placement? The pain of losing home and family, of moving into an unfamiliar environment, and the confusion of meeting an endless line of strange faces must be overwhelming. The person must also come to terms with her losses in physical and/or mental ability. We cannot begin to understand what it must be like.

Let us also consider where this person has come from. Is it from an acute hospital bed, where she has been through an endless barrage of tests and assessments; or after long months of fruitless rehabilitation; or from home, where she has finally been convinced that she or her family cannot 'cope' with her any more? For many, placement in nursing home care means finally admitting that there is no longer any hope of recovery.

Let us go one step further and consider how we, as workers in these centres, have greeted and introduced each new resident to their new home. I feel pangs of guilt as I do this, for I am reminded of the many times when I have become a little blasé about yet another new admission, and expected that person to settle into the home quickly and easily. (After all, they have been lucky to come to such a great nursing home!) How insensitive I have often been. Yet, for all the guilt I feel, I am reassured just a little by the fact that at least I did not greet each new person with still more tests, which only served to confirm their sense of failure and loss.

Staff need to offer a warm, caring, sensitive and undemanding environment to each new person to assist them through this time. Newly admitted residents need all the help they can get to regain some sense of a positive view of themselves and their new life. The last thing they need is yet more demoralising testing procedures.

The first responsibility of the extended care setting is to help each person integrate into the new 'home' environment. The new resident will need help to shake off that mental set of being the patient, dependent on the benevolent care of the hospital ward. Therefore, each person's introduction should be welcoming and positive, hinting at the possibilities of

239

a new, exciting phase in their life. An introduction which includes point-less testing procedures will simply confirm to new arrivals that they are yet again 'patients' in a different kind of hospital.

With this in mind, any assessment which is deemed necessary should be carried out as unobtrusively as possible to prevent further confusion and demoralisation.

A functional approach

The occupational therapist is trained to place every treatment technique into a functional, or practical, everyday setting. She is trained to focus on the positive existing abilities of a person, using them as a springboard to encourage development in the affected areas. Yet in many cases the as-sessment procedures which are available are totally removed from every-day experience. Many standard assessment procedures consist of puzzles, pen and paper tasks and questionnaires which are usually geared towards determining specific disorders, rather than discovering the remaining abili-ties of the person. They can be confusing and demoralising, pinpointing yet more areas of inability and loss. They can also seem pointless to the person being assessed, as they do not relate directly to the personal needs and circumstances of the client.

The assessment procedures used by occupational therapists should be functional and relevant to the client's needs. In any setting, an assessment should aim to discover the client's potential abilities, and find out what he or she wants to achieve through therapy. This is even more important in the extended care setting. The therapist must make sure that the assess-ment procedures do not intrude upon the lifestyle and emotional status of the client. The assessments should seek to find out how best to help that person to lead a fulfilling and rewarding life within the home. Therefore, observational assessment procedures are really the only appropriate form of assessment for the nursing home environment.

Purpose of assessment

It is important to establish the purpose of the assessment. What do we want to find out? Why do we need to know it? There is no point in submitting people to assessment without a clear purpose.

Appropriate placement

There are a number of reasons for assessment. One may be to determine suitable placement. The mental, physical and functional abilities, as well as the personal preferences and social circumstances of the person, need to be assessed accurately to ensure appropriate placement. This should have occurred before arrival at the nursing home or hostel. If it has not, then unobtrusive observation of the new resident in various activities will help to determine if he or she has been appropriately placed or could possibly manage in a more independent setting.

Causes of confusion

Assessment may also be necessary to discover the cause of confusion whether it is dementia, depression with disturbances in thinking, depression alone, or an acute medical problem. This will help to direct carers to the intervention needed to reverse or control the condition. This process can be assisted by assessments which observe the rate of deterioration of the client.

Program planning

However, the main purpose of assessment in the nursing-home environment will be to direct the planning of the activity program, so that it suits the interests and abilities of participants. Then it is working towards the main aim of improving the quality of life of the residents of the centre.

A recreational survey may be useful here to record information about the resident's past and present interests, and the lifestyle he or she has been used to. This will help to discover the best approach for the client's needs. The Queen Elizabeth Centre in Ballarat uses a Socialisation Assessment form to guide the collection of data (see p. 242). The information can be collected through casual chats with each individual. An alternative format for a social history is also included later in the chapter (p. 250).

Valid assessment tools

There are several assessment tools available to collect the information required. They are valid, reliable, observational assessments, which fulfil the purposes described above.

Alzheimer's disease and other forms of dementia

There are two observational assessment procedures worth noting.

The Rapid Disability Rating Scale[1] is a valid, reliable, observational assessment which indicates the rate of decline in functional abilities. It looks at all levels of functioning in the areas of activities of daily living, communication, confusion and depression, by making some very simple observations of the person's abilities and behaviour. This rating scale can help to discover the likely causes of deterioration, and can be used to assess the effectiveness of the course of intervention taken. Any carer can unobtrusively record results after only one training session.

The Functional Assessment Stage (FAST)[2] procedure enables the identification of at least 11 stages of Alzheimer's disease. Characteristics of change are described in functional terms, which can be observed without

242A WEALTH OF EXPERIENCE

SOCIALISATION ASSESSMENT

THE QUEEN ELIZABETH CENTRE, BALLARAT

U.R.NO: .... WARD: ....
SURNAME: .... GIVEN NAMES: ....
PAST ADDRESS: ....
....
D.O.B.: .... AGE: ....
PAST OCCUPATION: ....
MAJOR PROBLEMS: ....
DATE OF ASSESSMENT: ....

PHYSICAL DISABILITIES

- [ ] use of both arms
- [ ] use of one arm only
- [ ] — left arm
- [ ] — right arm

Special note: i.e. degree of disability ....
....

MENTAL STATUS

- [ ] alert [ ] forgetful [ ] wanders
- [ ] withdrawn [ ] other (specify): ....

ENDURANCE LEVEL

Activity sessions should be: [ ] short [ ] ½ day [ ] whole day
Outings should be: [ ] short [ ] ½ day [ ] whole day

COMMUNICATION ABILITY

able to speak: [ ] yes [ ] no
understands speech: [ ] yes [ ] no
able to write: [ ] yes [ ] no
able to read: [ ] yes [ ] no
  If yes, state whether [ ] normal print
                        [ ] large print

EYESIGHT

- [ ] normal [ ] wears glasses
- [ ] limited i.e. cataracts
able to watch television [ ] yes [ ] no

HEARING

- [ ] normal [ ] wears aid
- [ ] poor with aid [ ] poor without aid

MOBILITY

- [ ] walks unaided [ ] needs supervision
- [ ] walks with aid (specify):
- [ ] uses wheelchair all the time
- [ ] uses wheelchair for off-ward activities

Any precautions: (specify) ....
....

TRANSPORT

- [ ] bus [ ] car [ ] transfers to front seat
                    [ ] transfers to back seat
- [ ] maxi-taxi only

Special notes: ....
....

TOILETING

- [ ] independent (takes self to toilet)
- [ ] needs assistance [ ] needs transferring
- [ ] incontinent [ ] continent

Special notes: ....
....

DIET

- [ ] normal [ ] diabetic
- [ ] other (specify): ....

INTERESTS (past and present — refer back

of sheet): ....
....
Special comments: ....
....
....

* Used with permission from QEC, B.

(Tick appropriate boxes √)

Past interests

- [ ] Art — painting
- [ ] Bingo
- [ ] Cards
- [ ] Ceramics
- [ ] Clubs — Lodges, CWA, church groups, etc.
- [ ] Community service — Rotary, Council, etc.
- [ ] Cooking
- [ ] Crosswords
- [ ] Crafts — list main ones ....
  ....
- [ ] Dancing
- [ ] Drama
- [ ] Dining out
- [ ] Entertaining
- [ ] Fashion
- [ ] Films

- [ ] Floral work
- [ ] Gardening
- [ ] Games — chess, draughts, etc.
- [ ] Jigsaws
- [ ] Music — classical, choral work, bands, listening, played instrument?
- [ ] Photography
- [ ] Politics
- [ ] Pottery
- [ ] Picnics
- [ ] Radio
- [ ] Reading
- [ ] Religious activities — Church
- [ ] Television
- [ ] Travel — visiting places of interest
- [ ] Stamp/coin collecting
- [ ] Sports — played football, cricket, basketball, tennis
- [ ] Woodwork
- [ ] Writing letters

Activities resident may be interested in:............................
....

- [ ] Indoor bowling
- [ ] Community singing
- [ ] Music — classical
- [ ]   — other types
- [ ] Exercise to music
- [ ] Painting — oil and water colours
- [ ] Ceramics — moulded hobby
- [ ] Pottery
- [ ] Stamp/coin collecting
- [ ] Gardening
- [ ] Reading
- [ ] Crosswords — word games
- [ ] Cooking
- [ ] Cards — euchre, 500, crib, others
- [ ] Jigsaws
- [ ] Bingo

- [ ] Board games
- [ ] Group discussions
- [ ] Outings
  - [ ] day trips
  - [ ] counter lunch
  - [ ] to theatre
  - [ ] holidays
- [ ] Religious activities
- [ ] Films (type):............................
  ....
- [ ] Personal grooming
  — Nails and makeup
- [ ] Crafts
  - [ ] leatherwork
  - [ ] weaving
  - [ ] tapestry
  - [ ] pot pourri
  - [ ] woodwork
  - [ ] découpage
  - [ ] card making
  - [ ] paper making

disturbing the routine of the person being assessed. This observational assessment will help in the diagnosis of Alzheimer's disease and monitor the rate of deterioration of the individual. The functional results will help carers to determine the level of assistance the person will require in various activities.

Depression

Where depression is considered a possible contributing factor, the Modified Beck Depression Inventory[3] can be used to help establish depths of depression. The person is asked to choose which of a number of statements best describes how they are feeling. For example: 'I feel like a failure' or 'I don't feel I am any worse than anyone else.' When used carefully this procedure not only assists in collecting valid data, but may also help the person being assessed to understand their feelings and share them with another trusted person. This kind of assessment is useful in determining the cause of deterioration in functional abilities.

'Mini Mental State'

If more specific mental status assessment is required, and a questionnaire is unavoidable, a quick method is the Mini Mental State[4] grading, which is quite short. If the assessor does not push for answers when difficulties arise, it can be used without causing too much discomfort to the person being assessed. It is a valid test with scores that can discriminate between dementia, depression and acute conditions. The person being assessed can then be treated appropriately. This is important in cases where depression or an acute condition may otherwise be misdiagnosed as irreversible dementia, and a person requiring simple, appropriate intervention may go untreated.

However, the Mini Mental State grading must be used with discretion, and only in cases where other observational assessments have not produced a clear picture, and where misdiagnosis seems evident. It should not be used indiscriminately with everyone.

All these ratings allow the assessor to structure the gathering and recording process more consistently, particularly for research purposes, and to observe changes in functional abilities. For example, they may be useful in researching the effectiveness of various treatment programs aimed at improving the mental status of the participants. (There is also a variety of validated 'Activities of Daily Living' assessments available which can help in this type of research.[5]) However, the purpose of any assessment must be clear; it should definitely not be used indiscriminately, and where possible the person being assessed should understand the reason for the assessment. I cannot stress sufficiently the need to select observational assessment procedures in preference to formal testing, wherever possible.

The actual record sheets for these scales are not included here, as they should only be used with appropriate training and careful application. (Refer to the end of this chapter for further reading; see also Appendix B for staff development information, where further training options may be available.)

An observational recording system

I would like to propose a format for recording observations that can help specifically to determine the functional abilities of the residents (see p. 247). This format is not validated for research or diagnostic purposes, but it does provide a good base for recording information and produces a comprehensive profile of the needs and potential abilities of each individual. A program of activities which considers their needs and interests can then be devised with each resident.

How to use this record

Casual approach

The information for this record is collected in a number of ways. For example:

- through many casual chats, both individually with the person concerned, and in groups with other residents
- by helping the person to get up in the morning and prepare for the day
- by eating a meal with them
- by inviting them to join in a variety of activities, relevant to their interests and past experience, and observing their ability to participate (care should be taken to avoid causing too much frustration and failure)

Take time

Don't rush the collection of the information. Remember, the aim of recording the data is to discover the best ways to help that person improve their quality of life. Its collection should always stem from positive contacts with the person so that, if he or she dies before the record is complete, the process of assessment itself will have been a pleasurable, relevant and enriching time for that person. The assessment procedure will have already achieved its aim of improving quality of life.

Team approach

Close communication with the physiotherapy, nursing, domestic and administrative staff is essential to develop a full picture of the resident's abilities and interests. The responsibility of the occupational therapist is to record accurately the observations made, to interpret the information appropriately for program planning, and to keep the rest of the team up-to-date with any relevant findings and changes over time.

An example of the observational assessment process

The individual is invited to join a small group to cook and eat a meal together. In this setting the occupational therapist can observe the person's ability to participate in the following areas:

- social interactions with staff and other residents
- participation level and factors that affect it — mood; mental ability; physical ability; hearing; eyesight
- orientation — understanding of tasks/place/time
- memory: long-term memory — by observing the person's application of previous experience to the present cooking situation; short-term memory — ability to follow steps and maintain attention to task
- intellectual skills — in reading the recipe and in its application
- constructional skills — in the handling and appropriate use of utensils
- initiative — in volunteering assistance, advice or direction to others
- upper limb strength — in chopping, lifting and mixing
- mobility — in moving from table to cooker, to shelves, etc
- food preferences — the person's likes and dislikes revealed through discussions together; sense of taste and smell
- eating skills — is assistance required?

Documentation: A guide for a activity workers

Having described the assessment process for the occupational therapist, it is important to also identify the level of documentation and assessment that is appropriate for untrained activity staff. It is important that activity workers have access to an occupational therapist to assist them in establishing and maintaining their records.

The focus of assessment

1. Social and recreational histories should be available so the activity program can be designed to cater for the personality, needs and interests of each individual resident.
2. Observational assessment occurs continuously to determine:
   - the range of interests of the resident
   - the resident's willingness to participate in individual activities and social groups
   - the factors that limit participation in chosen activities (this may require OT consultation)

AN OCCUPATIONAL THERAPY
RECORD FOR OBSERVATIONAL ASSESSMENT

This record aims to provide a guide to discussions, and pointers to look for while observing the resident's participation in activities. It also offers a format to record the gathered information at the completion of the sessions. All comments should be brief.

1. GENERAL INFORMATION
Name:. . . . .

Places of residence throughout life: . . . .

Work history: . . . .

Interests/hobbies, past and present: . . . .

Likes/dislikes: . . . .

Significant life experiences: (That are freely offered). . . . .

2. PSYCHOLOGICAL STATUS/SOCIAL ABILITIES
Note any hearing loss: . . . .

Affect: (Signs of depression/zest for life) . . . .

Responsiveness/awareness of others:. . . . .

Level of integration with other residents:. . . . .

Appropriateness of conversational content:. . . . .

Use of nonverbal cues/ability to interpret them in others:. . . . .

3. MENTAL STATUS:
Indications of A. Orientation and confusion . . . .

B. Memory loss:stm/ltm . . . .

C. Intellectual abilities. . . . .

D. Constructional skills . . . .

E. Initiative . . . .

F. Ability to exercise choice/control of lifestyle (as demonstrated in conversations and activities) . . . .

4. PHYSICAL FUNCTION:
A. *Medical diagnosis:*. . . . .

B. *Mobility:* Independent/stick/wheelchair; assistance required: . . . .

C. *Upper limb strength:* (Note stiffness, dexterity, and steadiness of movements. Observe use of scissors, manipulative skills in activities, strength in throwing, carrying, mixing and lifting objects.) . . . . . .

D. *Transfers:* From bed to chair, toilet to chair, and into car. Type of assistance and transfer technique required:. . . . .

E. *Sensation:* Visual acuity (glasses), hearing (hearing aid), touch, movement, taste, smell:. . . . .

5. LEVEL OF INDEPENDENCE:
Toilet: Aids and assistance required, frequency of need: . . . .

Shower: Aids and assistance required:. . . . .

Dressing: Aids and assistance required:. . . . .

Grooming: Preference for hair care, makeup, manicure, shaving: . . . .

Eating: Aids, assistance required, special food needs, likes/dislikes:. . . . .

Outings: Transfer into car/bus; toilet needs. . . . .

Activities: Level of assistance required: share task; perform entire task unassisted. Personal preferences.

6. RESIDENT'S VIEW OF NURSING HOME PLACEMENT:
Include expectations, hopes for the future, indications of learned helplessness, perceptions of predictability and personal control over their environment. Desired level of participation in activities; preference for peaceful, individual activities, or for social contacts and group activity.

7. INDIVIDUAL PROJECTS:

8. GROUPS TO PARTICIPATE IN:

9. PROGRESS: New interest areas, level of independence and participation.

3 If an individual requires assistance to maintain independence in activities of daily living and to participate in other activities, the OT should be consulted to design a specific plan. The OT will then review the plan with the activity worker as required.

Assessment will occur in the following ways

1. Through many casual chats with the resident.
2. Through discussions with other team members.
3. By collecting a summary of the social history from the resident file, the resident and his or her relatives. (A comprehensive social history should already be available as part of standard admission procedures.) See Socialisation Assessment form (p. 242).
4. By involving residents in group and individual activities to observe each individual's ability to participate in their chosen activities.
5. OT assessment as required. For example, to assess whether intervention is required re maintenance of independence, activity adaptation, cognitive deficits or behavioural and social difficulties.

Recording findings

1. The activity worker will design a program to cater for the individual's needs. To do this, the activity worker should keep brief notes that include:
   - social summary that identifies the major focuses of the person's life
   - interests, activity ideas, etc
   - an Activity Plan that responds to the above
   - interventions specified by the OT
   - review comments

   All of the above can be recorded in a small card file. Keep notes brief so that they fit on one card. Add cards as needed to accommodate ongoing review comments. The OT can oversee this planning process, particularly where specific interventions are required.
2. Enter a brief summary into the Resident Care Plan. This information will then be available for nurses to implement at other times.
3. Record activity participation in the record books kept by the activity worker. Indicate the nature of the activity, the time spent and whether it is a group or individual session. This is the best form of record, as staff can see, at a glance, who is benefiting from the program and who is being overlooked. It also enables other staff to quickly see the range of activities being offered. The OT can instantly see if the prescribed activity plan matches the actual program. An Accounts book is ideal for this.

For example:

Name:	Monday		Tuesday		Wednesday		Thursday	
	Group	Indiv	Group	Indiv	Group	Indiv	Group	Indiv
Hardy, Joan	cooking 40 min		news discussion 20 min		Mass 30 min			
Thatcher, Daisy	cooking 40 min						painting 60 min	
Bloggs, Joe		music apprec			Mass 30 min			reminisce 15 min

4. The activity worker will constantly review the needs of residents and make appropriate changes to the program. She cannot, however, be expected to document every change in the program, but she will want to indicate to other staff any changes in the resident's level of function. The staff member responsible for global reporting can then enter these observations as part of the general comments.

   The activity worker may want to review the activity plans listed in the card file every now and then. This will help to keep the activities varied and appropriate. It can also help to revitalise the program if it is becoming stale or routine, as it is a permanent list of good activity ideas.

5. Ideally a 'This is Your Life' book will be compiled for residents with memory loss, and with those others who would like to compile a personal history for themselves. (It requires cooperation and help from many sources. It could be a great small group activity.)

Evaluation of the Activity Programs

At regular intervals, the OT can work with the activity staff to review the overall program — matching the activity plans with the record books and suggesting changes as necessary.

Social History

The importance of an accurate knowledge of each person's history cannot be over-emphasised. Consider the things that are important to you and what you would like staff to know about you if you found yourself in their care in the future. For example, recognition of the important achievements of your life; the food and drinks you like and dislike; the time you go to bed; your favourite television programs; your need for privacy or company; lifelong habits and rituals which give your day meaning. Such knowledge is important not simply so that you can continue to maintain these habits, but also so that you can be recognised as a valuable person who has lived a full life with a rich history of interesting stories and events.

SOCIAL HISTORY FORMAT

Dear .... , please take some time to complete this form as it will provide staff with a valuable tool to relate more meaningfully with your relative. This information will help staff to recognise your relative as a person with a full and active past. Of course it is up to you how much you want to let us know.

Mr/Mrs/Miss .... Childhood surname .... Preferred name ....

Date and place of birth .... Nationality.........................

First language spoken .... other ....

Religion ....

Time lived in Australia ....

Where did person spend most time as child? .... As adult? ....

Family History

Name of parents and occupations if known ....

Mother .... Father ....

Names of brothers and sisters in order of age (note if deceased) ....

....

Education — Schools ....

Higher education.................... Level achieved................................

Former Occupations ....

....

War service ....

Name of spouse (note if deceased) ....

Date and place of marriage...

Names of children in order of age (include spouses) ....

....

Names of grandchildren and great grandchildren ....

....

Please note work roles as relevant

Names of past pets ....

Names of special friends ....

Sporting interests...

Past hobbies/skills/interests/leisure activities ....

Present skills and interests ....

Favourite music (jazz, classical, opera, general) ....

Favourite TV and radio stations/programs ....

Reading preferences (books, magazines, newspapers)................................

Other relevant interests (please circle): gardening, cooking, church, painting, cards, fishing, craft, picnics, walks, table games, politics, shopping, knitting, films/videos, housekeeping, crosswords, puzzles, social outings: ballet, theatre, cinema, concerts, art gallery, museum, pub, restaurants, coffee shop. Specify details e.g. table games — monopoly, chess. Type of films — musicals, comedy, etc.........................

....

Favourite foods ....

Food dislikes ....

Shower or bathing preferences ....

Personality: has your relative usually been a very outgoing and sociable person or one who prefers the company of just a few close friends? Was he/she always a busy active person, or a quieter, more passive person in the past? (This information will help in the selection of group and/or individual activities) ....

....

Important life events: achievements, holidays, overseas trips, special memories (approximate dates would be helpful) ....

....

.... (use the back of the form if more space is required)

Any other information..

....

....

Thankyou for your cooperation.

The things which I would want staff to know about me, about my habits, my achievements and about my family would fill a few pages but I wonder how much we really know about the people who are presently in our care. Even such basic things as the way one prefers to shower. Adriana Tiziana, from the Alzheimer's Society told me of an Asian woman who panicked whenever she was taken to the shower. The confined steamy box shared with someone in a uniform triggered horrific images for her. Finally, after talking with her family, she was given a bucket and ladle to wash herself in the privacy of a large bathroom and she no longer refused to wash. There are no doubt many reasons why people, particularly if they have dementia, react negatively to certain activities within the nursing home, and this makes it important to acquire as much information as possible in order to know the best way to approach certain tasks with an individual.

It is not enough to rely on the knowledge that certain staff may collect about each person. All staff need to know about the individual characteristics of residents. This can only happen if a social history record is available for staff to refer to.

Opposite is a Social History Format which is useful to give to relatives of those residents who cannot provide accurate information for themselves. I have found that it is an invaluable tool for planning activities. Working as a consultant to nursing homes, I often assess and plan programs for residents whom I have little time to get to know. The presence of a social history makes a world of difference to the level of variety, interest and relevance of each resident's program plan. It can then be used to compile a 'This is Your Life' photo album with photographs and historical notes throughout, to help the person reflect upon and value their past life. Relatives could work on the album together with residents, or it could become a school history project for a student.

This format has been drawn from many sources including the Uniting Church Lodge program (which may have copied the idea from someone else), and other workers* who have since adapted it. Plenty of space should be left after each question to encourage detailed answers.

Some sample individual activity plans

Below are some examples of how information from a social history and knowledge of the physical capabilities of a resident can be used to develop more responsive activities. Information is drawn from social and medical histories, from talking with staff and from an assessment. It has been summarised to give a brief picture of each person and their individual

---

* Roz Hill devised this last version for Ashleigh Lodge Private Nursing Home in Melbourne.

activity plan. (Although based on a mixture of real people, names and details have been altered to protect identities.)

Frail gentleman with multi infarct dementia

Date: 4.8.94   **Resident:** Alfred Smith   **Date of Birth:** 12.3. 1912

Diagnosis: Subdural haematoma, transitory ischaemic attacks, multi infarct dementia, osteoarthritis.

Social summary: Married gentleman, who was a manager of a company and travelled a great deal. His wife is still active and continues to travel overseas now and again. He has 3 children who visit regularly. Alfred has always been very active, social and fun loving and had a successful working career.

Recreational interests: Past interests included gardening, cards, wood carving, crosswords, ballet, cinema, restaurants and other social outings, table tennis and shooting. He also enjoyed overseas travel, tennis, bowls, cricket and singing. He was a choir boy and played the piano.

Physical function: Confined to a wheelchair, needing assistance of one staff to transfer; left upper limb weakness but still functional; needs full assistance with toileting and needs padding and careful continence programming.

Psychological and intellectual function: He has decreased comprehension and while able to respond appropriately to simple conversation, he has difficulty initiating conversation and has limited speech content. He is however, a charming man who communicates much with his smile.

Activities of daily living: While he needs much assistance and supervision, he should be encouraged to assist with his personal care tasks where possible.

Meals: He needs prompting, careful positioning and his food cut up.

Recommendations

General activities: Alfred will join in day room activities but prefers practical activities. He may enjoy assisting the gardening group with simple potting tasks, cooking, simple woodwork tasks, e.g. sanding and painting a garden box or outdoor setting.

Men's club: A club atmosphere could be established for a few men who could share dinners, woodwork, cards and gambling games together. They may wish to plan some outings to various exhibitions relevant to their interests. The group may enjoy lunch at the pub, visiting a car exhibition, war memorials or other venues, watching videos together at night with a beer or two. A film buffs group could also be established.

Music: As Alfred is particularly musical he should have a chance to join the various musical activities at the home and to potter at the piano. He sings popular songs without difficulty.

Reminiscence: As he has had such an interesting life he needs opportunity to reflect upon and value his past achievements. A life history photo album would be ideal for him, so staff and visitors could look through it and affirm his past. His family could compile the album with Alfred during their visits or work on it at home.

Alert, visually impaired frail woman

Date: 4.8.94 **Resident:** Barbara Jones **Date of birth:** 10.11.1904
Diagnosis: Chronic congestive failure, non insulin dependent diabetes, visual impairment.

Social summary: Widowed with no children but has a supportive niece and friends. Barbara is an astute, humorous woman with highly developed social skills, but she prefers the company of a few friends and staff. She has developed a great friendship with her room mate, Jane, and they have a settled daily routine in their room. She is a very determined woman with a strong sense of her own wishes. She ran her own bakery business; her husband was a tradesman.

Recreational interests: Her past interests included pets, especially dogs, horse racing, chocolates, music, socialising with friends and shopping. She was an active auxiliary member.

Physical function: Barbara walks with a frame and supervision; requires assistance to transfer; adequate upper limb strength and function; can only see shadows so needs verbal cueing to direct her to objects and clothing, to position and describe her food and to assist her with mobility.

Psychological and intellectual function: While prone to depression due to her reducing independence and circumstances, Barbara is a very intelligent and alert woman with a great sense of humour. She enjoys visitors and the opportunity to chat about a whole range of topics.

Activities of daily living: Barbara will assist wherever she can with encouragement and assistance as required.

Meals: Food needs to be positioned carefully and described to Barbara. She may prefer a slightly deeper crockery plate to ensure that food does not slip away.

Recommendations

General activities: Barbara is content to remain in her room with Jane and to receive visitors regularly. She declines going out or joining any group activities. Activities which do occur need to be focused around the shared space of Jane and Barbara. They presently select the time of day that they prefer to listen to music and have established other routines which help to pass the time. She should however be kept informed of other activities and be invited to attend special events.

School tutorship: As Barbara enjoys visitors she would be an ideal person to link with a student who may like to produce a history, writing or poetry project with her. She could offer a student great assistance while gaining the pleasure of developing new friendships at the nursing home.

Dinners: Barbara and Jane both have some great friends with whom they might like to share special dinners. A table could be set up in their room for daily meals which would not only improve the social setting for Barbara and Jane but also enable then to entertain guests on a regular basis. A tablecloth, flowers, candles and chocolates would create a wonderful social atmosphere in their room.

Activities of daily living: Barbara is very keen to maintain her present level of independence; staff will need to give her time to take charge of her own personal care activities.

Social skills: As Barbara is prone to depression, her social skills need to be maintained and although her friendship with Jane is important to this, staff will need to offer regular social times to ensure that Barbara gains the social and intellectual stimulation that she needs.

Frail woman with moderate dementia

Data: 22.7.94   **Resident:** Francis Baker   **Date of birth:** 8.5.1904

Diagnosis: Increasing dementia, with decreased short and long-term memory. Fractured pelvis in 1992, bilateral cataracts.

Social summary: Francis is a widow, who was born in England but has spent many years in Australia. She has had a number of trips back to England and has many and varied interests.

Recreational interests: While her main interest has always been in her family, she has enjoyed cooking, walking, cards, monopoly, reading, especially books on history, geography, travel and biographies. She also liked gardening, shopping, musical comedy, cinema and ballet.

Physical function: Continent with prompting; walks with frame; adequate upper limb strength and function; decreased but functional hearing; wears glasses.

Psychological and intellectual function: Francis' memory loss, comprehension and confusion is gradually increasing. She is prone to Sundown distress and needs reassurance and attention at these times. She enjoys discussing her past and family, however she needs an informed listener to prompt her.

Activities of daily living: Needs supervision and some assistance with personal care. She is likely to need increasing levels of supervision but should be encouraged to do as much as she can herself. She eats without assistance.

Recommendations

General activities: As Francis is an active participant in most day room activities she is gaining opportunities to socialise and to maintain her physical mobility. This should continue to be encouraged. She enjoys music and most other day room activities.

Life record album: Francis would benefit if her social history were compiled into album form to help her talk about her life and family — which she obviously enjoys. Her family may like to make this a project to work on together with Francis at their visits, seeing it as a chance to organise, reflect upon and value her life together.

Outings: Francis should be encouraged to continue to go out regularly. Especially to galleries and musical events such as Morning Melodies at the Concert Hall and other local entertainment.

Dinners: Francis will enjoy special social dinners held within and outside the home, with other residents and relatives. She and a number of other women could select a relative to invite for dinner, then go shopping to buy the food, cook the meal and share it with their families.

ADL: All effort should be made to encourage Francis to maintain her present level of independence offering only supervision as needed to prevent confusion or discouragement. If her clothes are laid out in careful order she may maintain her automatic dressing skills for some time.

Eating: As Francis enjoys curries and Chinese food she should have the opportunity to eat out, participate in national cultural days, call in take-away Asian foods etc.

Other activities: Francis' extensive range of past interests can be drawn upon in many ways, from travel book discussions, or a regular world travel group which visits a different country each week, to looking at culture, food, artefacts, books etc. Staff from various cultures, or who have travelled, could assist or a volunteer could help out.

Music: Her interest in music should be channelled into regular music appreciation and percussion groups.

Sundown distress: She may benefit from joining a small group between 4 and 5pm. The group could go for a walk, have a late afternoon tea or play simple games and listen to relaxing music to assist them through this unsettled period.

Frail older gentleman

Date: 22.7.94 **Resident:** Joe Banner **Date of birth:** 5.11.1903
Diagnosis: Depression, hypertension, emphysema.
Social summary: Widowed, with a son who lives interstate. A granddaughter lives locally. He worked as a swimming teacher for a secondary

school for many years. He has great pride in his achievements with his students over that time. He has always preferred the company of just a few friends.

Recreational interests: Joe once enjoyed swimming, gardening, watching sports, reading and television. He now reports that he has very little interest in anything but television.

Physical function: Joe can only walk with physiotherapy assistance and is otherwise confined to a wheelchair and due to his apathy will often not assist to weight bear when being attended by staff. He is generally frail with poor strength and little motivation to help himself. He is continent with careful control.

Psychological and intellectual function: Joe much prefers to stay in his room and watch TV. He has no desire to socialise, sometimes aggressively rejecting social contact altogether, but he will respond to the odd chat with staff. He is a reasonably alert man with a strong sense of what he does and does not want.

Activities of daily living: He needs full assistance with all areas of personal care and hygiene.

Meals: He eats independently if his food is carefully positioned.

Recommendation

Social isolation: Joe will talk to staff and visitors about his teaching years and enjoys a brief chat. It would be worth collecting some old year books, old school magazines and other school memorabilia for Joe to look through. Maybe a community visitor, who attended Joe's school, could visit regularly. The material could be compiled into a life history album. This would provide some positive material for short regular chats.

Conclusion

By using the occupational therapist's comprehensive knowledge in the areas of higher cortical function, physical function, and mental, emotional and social functioning, appropriate information can be derived from this observational approach. It will enable more realistic treatment planning and goal setting for each individual's therapy or activity program. At the same time, it refrains from using testing procedures which expose more areas of failure and inability to the person being tested. Where diagnosis or research is required in the extended care setting, those valid assessment procedures which are observational in nature should always be used in preference to intrusive testing procedures. In this way, necessary data can be collected without detracting from the creation of a warm, homelike environment or the lifestyle of the residents.

References

1. Linn MW, Linn BS. The Rapid Disability Rating Scale. *Journal of the American Geriatric Society.* 1982; 30(6):378.

2. Reisberg B. Ferris SH, De Leon MJ. Senile dementia of the Alzheimer type: Diagnostic and differential diagnostic features with special reference to functional assessment staging. In J Triber, WH Gispen, eds. *Senile Dementia of the Alzheimer Type,* 1985.

3. Beck AT, Ward CH, Mendelson M, Mock J, Erbaugh J. An inventory for measuring depression. *Archives of General Psychiatry.* 1961; 4:53–63.

4. Folstein MF, Folstein S, McHugh PR. A practical method for grading the cognitive state of patients for the clinician. *Journal of Psychiatric Research.* 1975; 12:189–198.

5. Kane RA, Kane RL. *Assessing the Elderly: A Practical Guide to Measurement.* Lexington, MA: Lexington Books, 1981. Very useful reading.

Chapter 18
A Step-by-Step Approach to Activities

Mary loved gardening but a stroke had left her confined to a wheelchair and without the use of her left hand. The garden beds at the centre seemed so far out of her reach. Long-handled tools helped a little, but they really required the use of two hands to gain adequate control over them. The garden club came up with a solution. It redesigned the section of the garden that was overlooked by the lounge area.

The garden here had a path going past a grassy embankment. The embankment was dug out and replaced with a raised garden bed bordered with sleepers. With other interested residents, Mary could wheel her chair close to the bed and pull weeds, plant seedlings and prune the small shrubs without any difficulty. In some cases, where two hands were needed, she would work with another resident.

The garden bed provided a very attractive view for the lounge area, one of which everyone felt most proud.

Adapting activities

Except where physical and mental disabilities are very severe, there should be some way of helping each person take part in the activities they enjoy. As Mary's story indicates, it may require only some simple observations of the abilities of the person concerned, and the nature of the task, to discover a solution to the presenting difficulties.

This chapter discusses the process required to adapt activities to the appropriate level of the participants. The assessment phase already described in Chapter 17 is the first step in this process. The abilities of each resident need to be assessed accurately to enable their involvement in their selected activities. Once the interests and abilities of the individuals are established, the next step is to break down the selected activity into its component parts, in order to match them to the abilities of each participant. This is known as activity analysis.

258

Activity analysis

In the therapy situation, an activity is often analysed to find out, for example, what demands it will place on the participant that will facilitate the return of a lost physical function. This may not be the main aim of activity analysis in the extended care setting. Instead of seeking a therapeutic outcome, the activity is analysed to develop ways in which a person can participate in a chosen pursuit. The aim is to help residents maintain an active involvement in the things they most enjoy. It may be either physical or mental limitations which make consideration of this process necessary. For example, one-handedness after a stroke or the presence of confusion may make it difficult to follow the logical sequence of steps required by some activities.

So an activity is broken down into its component parts to discover which steps in the activity are making it difficult for a person to participate fully. Alternative solutions can then be discussed with the resident. They may include:

- using an aid of some kind to stabilise or support the work
- positioning equipment and participant in the way that best assists performance of the task
- simplifying the requirements and offering supervision for confused participants
- seeking assistance from another resident or volunteer to perform certain steps of the activity with the resident
- looking at variations in the nature of the task

If a thorough analysis of the chosen activity indicates that the person cannot manage the task, alternative activities may need to be discussed.

The activity analysis may occur at the group or individual level. In the group, the activity can be broken into steps which are then matched to the ability of each resident. The team may achieve the final product together, or some members of the group may prefer to do the entire activity themselves. In this case, they may like to work alongside the other group members who are sharing the task. A flexible approach is most important.

In a group

An example may be the cooking group. The group decides to make chutney. Tasks include:

- the collection of ingredients and utensils
- the chopping of onions, tomatoes and other ingredients
- the measurement of ingredients and the addition of spices and liquids

- cooking, stirring and the decision that the chutney is cooked to perfection
- bottling, labelling, decorating and pricing

Group members can each be involved in every step as a team, or form a process line: one chopping onions, another tomatoes, another measuring, another stirring and supervising the cooking, while others bottle and label.

Participants can be involved at the level which interests them most and which best suits their abilities. For example, one may cut all the vegetables in half so that another person, with only one functional hand, can chop the pieces more easily. Another with better eyesight may read the recipe and do the measuring. Non-slip mats and one-handed utensils will assist others. Often individuals with some degree of dementia enjoy the chopping and stirring, yet cannot follow the recipe or measure ingredients. In the group setting, everyone gains the satisfaction of achieving the final product together.

For the individual

The same process can be applied at the individual level. A woman may enjoy tapestry work but, after her stroke and decline in eyesight, finds she is unable to engage in this occupation. The activity requires her to be able to thread a needle with fine threads, then to support the work with one hand while sewing with the other. Good eyesight is needed to discriminate between slight variations in colour, and to see the holes in the work. The completed piece needs to be framed or perhaps sewn onto a cushion.

Accurate eye hand coordination is needed to place the needle in the correct holes. She finds the fine holes and threads difficult to manipulate, so a larger block-style design is chosen which uses thick wools. The work is secured to a frame, which is clamped at an angle on the working surface. She may require some supervision at times; a friend, relative or volunteer may be able to assist. A needle-threading machine may help, or a volunteer could help by threading the needle and finishing off the final article.

Summary of steps required

1. Assess the interests and abilities of the participant.
2. Ask the participant to select the activity.
3. Determine the difficulties which are preventing successful involvement in the task.
4. Study the steps required to complete the task.
5. Note which of these steps the participant can or cannot perform successfully.

6. Consider the options of a team approach or individual work.

7. Research the availability of aids which may assist the task. (The Independent Living Centre, the Association of Occupational Therapists, a consultant occupational therapist, the School of Occupational Therapy or one of the Disability Information Bureaus may be able to advise you here. See Chapter 9 and Appendices A and B.)

8. Determine the degree of supervision required; skilled or voluntary?

9. Discuss with the participant which approach she would prefer to use in order to do the activity.

10. Take care to work within the concentration span and frustration limits of that individual.

It may make all the difference

This process of analysis and matching of tasks may seem too obvious to address in this manner, but sometimes a person is deprived of an activity simply because this process has not been considered. Discussion with the resident, careful consideration of alternatives, some positive lateral thinking, and/or consultation with an occupational therapist may be all that is needed to enable the person to participate satisfactorily.

Chapter 19

Program Planning: A Summary

The overriding message for planning an activity program is that no program is worthwhile unless it is exactly what residents want and is based on careful discussion with the residents themselves. Yet it should also offer participants the option to try completely new experiences in addition to familiar ones. In this way, participants are given the chance to discover the areas that interest them most. The result will be a program which is creative, varied and responsive to the interests of all the participants.

However, there are many philosophical and structural considerations which must be observed to ensure that the program really does achieve its aim: to improve the quality of life of all the people who are in residence in an aged care facility. The requirements for this are summarised in this chapter.

A well designed program should occur if:

- assessment is occurring appropriately
- activities are adapted as necessary to ensure successful participation
- structures exist to ensure ongoing direction and feedback from residents and participants
- a sense of humour pervades throughout

The requirements

Assessment

Non-intrusive assessment of each individual's abilities, interests and social preferences should be ongoing (see Chapter 17).

Residents' committee

The residents' committee is essential to direct the program and gain feedback about preferred activities. The program should be planned *by* them, not *for* them. Active participation is then far more likely (see Chapter 2).

Team approach

The team starts with the resident and his or her family, and then includes all other staff and volunteers who are involved in the life of the individual. This team determines the program content together (see Chapter 2).

Program meetings

The members of the meeting, representing the various departments of the centre, gather round a yearly planner to suggest activities and events. All contribute ideas and are then aware of the requirements which will be made of them for the various events (see Chapter 2).

Yearly planner

A large planning calendar enables the activity organisers to gain a thorough overview of the range and regularity of activities and events. One can quickly assess if the program is really meeting the needs and requests of participants, or if it is becoming repetitive and catering for the needs of just a few (see Chapter 2).

Nature of the activities

The program will include regular daily, weekly and monthly activities, thus offering predictability to residents. It will also provide special events of a one-off nature. This enables the program to target the whole population of the centre, with its varied needs and interests (see Chapters 4, 5, 6 and 7).

Creative routine

Many of the special events can be slotted into the regular weekly program, and regular group times used to do the preparation activities for the special events. This helps to offer variety and purpose, without losing a sense of predictability. The routine can then be maintained without it becoming boring and restrictive. Most residents prefer a predictable routine; it helps to retain their sense of control over life events. However, having said this, be prepared to break the routine now and then to create a breath of fresh air — most people enjoy a change (see Chapters 4 and 5).

Group selection

Participant selection for group activities will reflect the interests, personalities and abilities of each individual. Friendships and personal preferences should also be respected (see Chapter 1).

Advertising

Residents need prior warning of the choices that are available to them so that they can actively choose which activities they will pursue. This is most important as it gives residents a sense of being in control of both the program itself and their participation in it (see Chapter 2).

Community involvement

Wherever possible, the resources within the local community should be drawn upon before establishing separate programs within the centre. Contact and involvement with people of all ages should be encouraged (see Chapters 9, 10, 11, 12 and 13).

To Conclude

The ideas presented in this book are designed to motivate workers in the field to take positive action now, to improve the quality of life of the residents at their particular centre. An activity program must be sufficiently creative and diverse to respond to the needs and interests of every resident, and must give people the option to participate or decline involvement in the selection of activities.

Workers must always remember that the main reason for the provision of activity programs is to create an environment in which all residents can exercise control over all aspects of their lives, in order to maintain their dignity and self-esteem. This is the key to ensuring that the programs really do enhance the quality of life of the participants.

Good planning will mean children and laughter are commonplace in a nursing home.

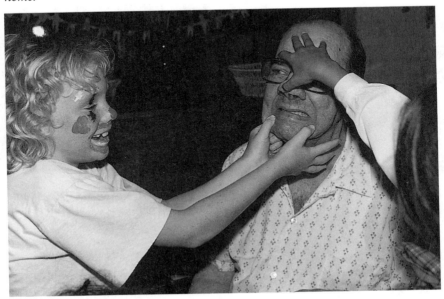

The older people in our community have every right to expect that their lives in old age can be as fulfilling as in earlier years, regardless of their disabilities and living circumstances. We shall be old one day, too. We need to invest in our own futures. While we have the power to act we must make sure that aged care facilities are of a high standard.

And remember, if the staff are enjoying themselves, the residents' level of care and enjoyment can only improve too. So go out and enjoy yourselves!

Appendix A
Information Services

Listed here are the various services and departments which may offer assistance in developing a resource file relevant to your centre's needs. The lists are not exhaustive but provide a starting point that will enable you to find information relevant to your particular area. The departments listed should be able to direct you to the local body whose services are required. Chapter 9 describes the various agencies in more depth and provides a guide to finding information.

The services in this appendix are listed under the following headings:

- Recreation
- Ageing
- Disability information services
- Art and entertainment resources
- Holidays and outings
- Volunteers centres
- Funding sources

Staff development and support organisations are listed in Appendix B; adult community education centres are listed in Appendix E.

Recreation

State Departments of Sport and Recreation

VIC: Sport and Recreation Victoria — A Portfolio of the Department of the Arts, Sport and Tourism, GPO Box 2392V, Melbourne VIC 3001. 123 Lonsdale Street, Melbourne Vic 3000. Tel: (03) 666 4200. Fax: (03) 666 4394.

NSW: Department of Sport, Recreation and Racing, PO Box 422, North Sydney NSW 2059. 1–5 Miller Street, North Sydney NSW 2060. Tel: (02) 923 4234. Fax: (02) 923 4345.

SA: Department of Sport and Recreation, GPO Box 1865, Adelaide SA 5000. Level 9, Citri Centre, 11 Hindmarsh Square, Adelaide SA 5001.

Tel: (08) 226 7301. Fax: (08) 226 7399.

QLD: Department of Tourism, Sport and Racing, Division of Sport and Recreation, GPO Box 26, Brisbane QLD 4001. 3rd Floor, 85 George Street, Brisbane QLD 4000. Tel: (07) 237 1268. Fax: (07) 237 9879.

WA: Ministry of Sport and Recreation, PO Box 66, Wembley WA 6014. 1st floor Penny Lakes Stadium, Meagher Dr, Floreat Park WA 6014. Tel: (09) 387 9700. Fax: (09) 387 9726.

TAS: Department of Tourism, Sport and Recreation, GPO Box 501E Hobart TAS 7001. Kirksway House, Kirksway Place, Battery Point, Hobart

7004. Tel: (002) 30 2748. Fax: (002) 23 7423.

ACT: ACT Office of Sport, Recreation and Racing, PO Box 1156, Tuggeranong ACT 2901. 1st floor, Centrepoint Building, Anketell Street, Tuggeranong ACT 2900. Tel: (06) 293 5643. Fax: (06) 293 5637.

NT: Office of Sport, Recreation and Ethnic affairs, GPO Box 1448, Darwin NT 0801. Tel: (089) 82 2311. Fax: (098) 81 5169.

Australian Letter Index in Recreation and Sport, Footscray Institute of Technology Library, PO Box 64, Footscray VIC 3011. Tel: (03) 688 4259.

'Life Be In It' Australia, 106 Batman Ave, Melbourne VIC 3004. Tel: (03) 654 8222.

Institute of Recreation, PO Box 287, Brunswick VIC 3065.

ACHPER (Australian Council for Health, Physical Education and Recreation) National Office: ACHPER Inc. 214 Port Road, Hindmarsh SA 5007. Tel: (08) 340 3388. Fax: (08) 340 3399.

ACT: PO Box 873, Civic Square, ACT 2608. Tel: (06) 207 3463. Fax: (06) 207 3179.

NSW: PO Box 84, Croydon NSW 2132. Tel: (02) 744 8221. Fax: (02) 744 6917.

QLD: PO Box 517, Mt Gravatt QLD 4122. Tel: (07) 849 4385. Fax: (07) 849 7191.

SA: Sturt Street, Adelaide SA 5000. Tel: (08) 213 0628. Fax: (08) 211 7115.

VIC: GPO Box 412C, Melbourne VIC 3001. Tel: (03) 887 8740. Fax: (03) 887 8740.

WA: PO Box 57, Claremont WA 6010. Tel: (09) 383 7708.

NT: PO Box 2331, Darwin NT 0801. Tel: (089) 81 5375. Fax: (089) 81 3890.

TAS: PO Box 166, Launceston TAS 7250. Tel: (003) 83 4353.

NICAN (National Information Communication and Awareness Network) **Inc,** PO Box 407, Curtin ACT 2605. Tel: (06) 285 4371 Toll Free 008 806 769.

Ageing

Council on the Ageing

National Executive Director: Council on the Ageing (Australia), 3rd floor, 464 St Kilda Road, Melbourne VIC 3004. Tel: (03) 820 2655. Fax: (03) 820 9886.

WA: Executive Director, Council on the Ageing (WA) Inc, 11 Freedman Road, Mount Lawley WA 6050. Tel: (09) 272 2133. Fax: (09) 370 1807.

SA: Executive Director, Council on the Ageing Inc, 45 Flinders Street, Adelaide SA 5000. Tel: (08) 232 0422. Fax: (08) 232 0433, 008 182 324, 018 835 439.

TAS: Administration Manager, Council on the Ageing (Tasmania) Inc, 2 St Johns Avenue, New Town TAS 7008. Tel: (002) 28 1897. Fax: (002) 28 0481.

VIC: Executive Director, Council on the Ageing (Victoria) Inc, 126 Wellington Parade, East Melbourne VIC 3002. Tel: (03) 416 0822. Fax: (03) 416 2829.

ACT: Executive Director, Council on the Ageing (ACT) Inc, Hughes Community Centre, Wisdom Street, Hughes ACT 2605. Tel: (06) 282 3422. Fax: (06) 285 3422.

NSW: Executive Director, Council on the Ageing (NSW) Inc, 34 Argyle Place, Millers Point NSW 2000. Tel: (02) 247 3388. Fax: (02) 247 4324.

QLD: Executive Director, Council on the Ageing (Queensland) Inc, Sir Leslie Wilson Youth Centre, Tenth Avenue, Windsor QLD 4030.

NT: Executive Director, Council on the Ageing (NT) Inc, 18 Bauhinia Street,

Nightcliff NT 0810. Tel: (089) 481 511. Fax: (089) 481 665.

Alzheimer Associations

VIC: 98 Riversdale Road, Hawthorn VIC 3122. Tel: (03) 818 3022, 008 182 209. Fax: (03) 818 3940.

NSW: PO Box 42, North Ryde NSW 2113. Tel: (02) 805 0100, 008 810 604. Fax: (02) 805 1665.

NT: PO Box 380919, Winnellie NT 0821. Tel: (089) 227 420. Fax: (02) 089 276 204.

QLD: PO Box 446, Lutwyche QLD 4030. Tel: (07) 857 4043, 008 017 212. Fax: (07) 857 3693.

SA: PO Box 202, Eastwood SA 5063. Tel: (08) 373 2670, 008 182 209. Fax: (08) 373 2675.

TAS: PO Box 1606, Hobart TAS 7001. Tel: (002) 34 8884. Fax: (002) 36 9012.

WA: PO Box 1099, Subiaco WA 6008. Tel: (09) 388 2800, 008 644 333. Fax: (09) 388 2739.

Disability Information Services

ACROD (Australian Council for Rehabilitation of the Disabled)

NSW: Executive Officer, ACROD NSW Division, 55 Charles Street, Ryde NSW 2112. Tel: (02) 809 4488. Fax: (02) 809 6517.

VIC: Executive Officer, ACROD VIC Division, PO Box 210, Hampton VIC 3188. Tel: (03) 597 0157. Fax: (03) 598 4158.

TAS: Executive Officer, ACROD TAS Division, Hampden House Community Centre, 82 Hampden Road, Battery Point TAS 7004. Tel: (002) 23 6086. Fax: (002) 23 6136.

QLD: Executive Officer, ACROD QLD Division, PO Box 101, Fortitude Valley Qld 4006. Tel: (07) 250 1511. Fax: (07) 252 3387.

ACT: Executive Officer, ACROD ACT Division, PO Box 29, Garran ACT 2605. Tel: (06) 282 4333. Fax: (06) 281 3488.

WA: Executive Officer, ACROD WA Division, PO Box 8136, Perth Business Centre, Perth WA 6849. Tel: (09) 222 2961. Fax: (09) 222 2963.

SA: ACROD SA Division, c/- Royal Society for the Blind of SA Inc, PO Box 196, Greenacres SA 5086. Tel: (08) 261 4611. Fax: (08) 266 3310.

NT: Alice Springs Disabled Persons Bureau, PO Box 721, Alice Springs NT 0870. Tel: (089) 515 882. Fax: (089) 515 884.

NT: Darwin HPA Inc, PO Box 37363, Darwin NT 0821. Tel: (089) 47 0681. Fax: (089) 84 4586.

Health, Housing and Community Services

PO Box 9848, Capital City. TEL: **VIC:** (03) 285 8888. **NSW:** (02) 225 3555. **WA:** (09) 426 3444. **SA:** (08) 237 6111. **ACT:** (06) 289 1555. **TAS:** (002) 211 4111. **NT:** (089) 463 444. **QLD:** (07) 360 2555.

Disabled Person's Information Bureau, 555 Collins Street, Melbourne VIC 3000. Tel: (03) 616 7704.

Independent Living Services

VIC: 52 Thistlethwaite Street, South Melbourne VIC 3205. Tel: (03) 254 5400.

NSW: 600 Victoria Road, Ryde NSW 2112. Tel: (02) 808 2233.

SA: 180 Daws Road, Daws Park SA 5041. Tel: (08) 276 3455.

QLD: ILC, c/- Ward 1, Repatriation Hospital, Newdegate Street, Greenslopes QLD 4120. Tel: (07) 394 7471.

WA: 3 Lemnos Street, Shenton Park WA 6008. Tel: (09) 382 2011.

ACT: ILC, 24 Parkinson Street, Western ACT 2611. Tel: (06) 205 1900.

Art and Entertainment Resources

Australian College of Entertainers (ACE) Promotions, 33 Bridpoint Street, South Melbourne VIC 3205. Tel: (03) 699 1355. A useful resource. Similar organisations will be found in other States.

Arts Access Society, 109–11 Sturt Street, South Melbourne VIC 3205. Tel: (03) 699 8299.

Victorian College of the Arts, 234 St Kilda Road, Melbourne VIC 3004. Tel: (03) 685 9300.

Playback Theatre. This is a group which involves the stories and experiences of the audience in their performance. The stories are enacted immediately. It is a very successful stimulus for reminiscing among older people (see Chapter 4). St Silas Hall, Bridpoint Street, South Melbourne VIC 3205. Tel: (03)690 9253.

Holidays and Outings

The tourist bureaus in each State can provide assistance for those travelling with special needs. The State Government Tourist Bureaus are particularly helpful.

RACV/Victorian Information Centre, 550 Princess Highway, Noble Park VIC 3174. Tel: (03) 790 3333. **Adelaide**: 16 Grenfell Street, Adelaide SA 5000. Tel: (08) 231 4129. **Sydney:** 403 George Street, Sydney NSW 2000. Tel: (02) 299 2288.

Tasmanian Travel Centres: Melbourne Tel: (03) 206 7933. Fax: (03) 650 4421. **Sydney** Tel: (02) 202 2033. Fax: (02) 202 2055. **Adelaide** Tel: (08) 400 5533. Fax: (08) 232 9108. **Brisbane** Tel: (07) 405 4133. Fax: (07) 405 4140. **Canberra** Tel: (06) 209 2133. Fax: (06) 209 2155.

South Australian Tourism Commission: 18 King William Street, Adelaide SA 5000. Tel: (08) 212 1505. **Melbourne** Tel: (03) 614 6522. **Sydney** Tel: (02) 232 8388. **Perth** Tel: (09) 481 1268.

Queensland Government Travel Centre: Corner Edward and Adelaide Streets, Brisbane QLD 4000. Tel: (07) 833 5337. **Melbourne** Tel: (03) 654 3866. **Sydney** Tel: (02) 232 1788. **ACT** Tel: (06) 248 8411. **Adelaide** Tel: (08) 212 2399. **Perth** Tel: (09) 322 1777.

NSW Travel Centres: GPO Box 7050, Sydney NSW 2001. Tel: (02) 231 4444. **Melbourne** Tel: (03) 670 7461. **Brisbane** Tel: (07) 229 8833. **Adelaide** Tel: (08) 231 3167.

Societies for the Disabled: Many societies have their own specialised holiday facilities available, designed for easy wheelchair access. Any of the Disability Information Services can direct you to the relevant body in your State. For example, in Victoria, the Yooralla Society has a caravan and campsite available for hire by groups with disabled members.

Yooralla Society of Victoria: Recreation Department, PO Box 88, South Melbourne VIC 3205. Tel: (03) 254 5666.

Bus Tours: All the major bus companies now have some buses with wheelchair facilities, which can usually be hired with a driver. Greyhound and Austfun are examples. Some companies, such as Cumalong Tours, run specialised tours for older people.

Cumalong Tours: PO Box 224, Northbridge NSW 2063. Tel: (02) 958 8379. Fax: (02) 958 8950. Although most of their individual tours are confined to NSW and Southern Victoria, they will run contract tours throughout Australia. They have smaller buses to enable groups to plan tours to suit their interests. In the future, Cumalong tours plans to expand its individual tours throughout Australia.

They provide full nursing care, assistance with meals, showering, toileting, mobility as needed; carry special equipment; offer varied, interesting and fun itineraries with modified activities according to disability levels. All tours are in modern, air-conditioned, fully accessible buses. Special programs are designed for older groups with an emphasis on sightseeing and passive pursuits, but they can be as active as required.

Holiday Associations: Various bodies exist in each State, such as the **Camping Association, Outdoor Education Association** and the **Host Farms Association,** which may offer some facilities accessible to the disabled. The Disability Information services or the tourist bureaus can be contacted for up-to-date details on these associations.

Volunteers Centres

The following centres offer support to volunteers and match volunteers to jobs through a job bank system. They also house resource libraries with information relevant to volunteers.

Volunteer Centre of Victoria: 247 Flinders Lane, Melbourne VIC 3000. Tel: (03) 650 5541.

Volunteer Centre of SA: 155 Pirie Street, Adelaide SA 5000. Tel: (08) 232 0199.

Volunteer Centre of NSW: Level 2, 105 Pitt Street, Sydney NSW 2000. Tel: (02) 231 4000.

Volunteer Centre of Qld: PO Box 623, Brisbane QLD 4001. 4th floor Penny Building, 155 Adelaide Street, Brisbane. Tel: (07) 209 9700.

Funding Sources

Trusts: *Philanthropic Trusts in Australia,* Australian Council of Educational Research Ltd, Radford House, Frederick Street, Hawthorn VIC 3122. (1983). This book outlines the various trust funds available throughout Australia. It gives a guide to preparing applications for grants, and classifies the trusts into their charitable purposes so that you can approach those trusts which are most likely to be favourable towards your field of work.

Government Funding and Information Services: Funding is often available through the Federal and State departments of Health and Community Services at various times. The funding arrangements vary from year to year. For example, in the past, Dementia Grants were available for the establishment of some programs. The various departments should be approached to discover the nature of grants available at any one time. These departments can often provide lists of community services and other information relevant to your centre's region of operation. The departments are listed in the government sections of the telephone directory.

Appendix B
Staff Development and Support Services

Staff Development Services

All staff should have opportunities to develop their skills in this important field so that older people receive expert care. The following centres offer a variety of valuable services.

Colleges of Health Sciences

The colleges listed below are the training campuses for the various paramedical applied science degree courses in Health Sciences. They also run other undergraduate and postgraduate courses which are relevant to aged care.

Cumberland College of Health Sciences, University of Sydney, PO Box 170, Lidcombe NSW 2141. East Street, Lidcombe NSW 2141. Tel: (02) 646 6444. Also offers and Associate Diploma of Diversional Therapy course.

University of South Australia, Faculty of Health and Biomedical Sciences. School of Occupational Therapy, PO Box 2471, Adelaide SA 5000. North Terrace, Adelaide SA 5000. Tel: (08) 302 2484.

University of Queensland, Department of Occupational Therapy, Therapies Building, St Lucia QLD 4072. Tel: (07) 365 2652; (07) 365 2820.

Curtin University of Technology (Perth), Schools of Therapy, Selby Street, Shenton Park WA 6008. Tel: 381 0600.

Edith Cowan University(WA), Claremont Campus, Goldsworthy Road, Claremont WA 6010. Tel: (09)383 0333.

Latrobe University, Carlton Campus, Locked Bag 12, Carlton South VIC 3053. 625 Swanston Street, Carlton VIC 3053. Tel: Occupational Therapy School (03) 285 5238.

Other training centres

Mayfield Centre 11–27 Mayfield Avenue, Malvern VIC 3144. Tel: (03) 822 3221. Offers a package called 'Activities for Quality of Life in Residential Care: A 24-part video training program for carers of frail elderly persons'. The program provides in-service on-site training which requires very little time to implement, while offering theoretical and practical understanding. It is suitable for all staff and interested relatives and visitors.

The package is designed to be viewed over a full year, to enable each aspect of the training program to be applied to the setting. It is both practical and educational. Each 8-week series is followed by an 8-week consolidation period, when videos are viewed again and implemented.

Topics cover program planning, volunteers, small group method, confusion and dementia, reality orientation and validation therapy, lifestyle, activity choices, implementing change. These topics are viewed alternately with electives which have a more practical focus and demonstrate the suggested activities.

Mayfield also offers short training courses for people planning to implement the package.

Centre for Social Health, PO Box 53, Fairfield VIC 3078. 1st floor, Yarra House, Fairfield Hospital, Yarra Bend Road, Fairfield VIC 3078. Tel: (03) 280 2948.

Carmel Hurst and Associates, 62 Seymour Road, Elsternwick VIC 3185. Tel: (03) 523 9418. Specialises in the provision of services in the area of aged care.

Staff Support Organisations

Peer and staff support is essential for maintenance of morale and to provide a wide-ranging resource of ideas exchange. There are various professional and purpose-based support groups established throughout Australia.

Australian Association of Occupational Therapists (AAOT), Federal Executive, 6 Spring Street, Fitzroy VIC 3065. Tel: (03) 416 1021. Fax (03) 416 1421.

Member Association State Secretaries

ACT: The Secretary, PO Box E171, Parkes ACT 2600. Tel: (06) 287 1644. Fax: (02) 287 1640.

NSW: The Secretary, PO Box 142, Ryde NSW 2112. Tel: (02) 807 1822. Fax: (02) 807 1609.

VIC: The Secretary, PO Box 143, Ashburton VIC 3147. Tel: (03) 885 0301. Fax: (03) 885 0302.

QLD: The Secretary, 30 Trevallyan Drive, Daisy Hill QLD 4127. Tel: (07) 208 1058. Fax: (07) 808 1640.

SA: The Secretary, PO Box 7006, Adelaide SA 5000. Tel: (08) 387 2870.

TAS: The Secretary, PO Box 531, Kingston TAS 7050. Tel: (002) 29 7763. Fax: (002) 29 7763.

WA: The Secretary, 4A/266 Hay Street, Subiaco WA 6008. Tel: (09) 388 1490. Fax (09) 388 1492.

NT: The Secretary, PO Box 41154, Casuarina NT 0811. Fax: (089) 227 482.

TARCRAQ National Office, PO Box 284, Zillmere QLD 4034. Tel: (07) 263 7677, 008 773 345.

NSW: TARCRAQ, PO Box 360, Randwick NSW 2031. Tel: (02) 314 5496.

Recreation

Institute of Recreation, PO Box 287, Brunswick VIC 3056.

ACHPER National Office, ACHPER Inc, 214 Port Road, Hindmarsh SA 5007. Tel: (08) 340 3388. Fax: (08) 340 3399.

Geriaction: Geriaction, Suite 401, 282 Victoria Avenue, Chatswood NSW 2067. Tel: (02) 412 2145 Fax: (02) 411 6618.

NSW: The Secretary Geriaction, Suite 401, 282 Victoria Avenue, Chatswood NSW 2067.

VIC: The Secretary Geriaction, PO Box 469, Hawthorn VIC 3122.

SA: The Secretary Geriaction, PO Box 160, Eastwood SA 5063.

WA: The Secretary Geriaction, PO Box 580, South Perth WA 6151.

TAS: The Secretary Geriaction, PO Box 380, Moonah TAS 7009.

QLD: The Secretary Geriaction, PO Box 687, Kenmore QLD 4069.

Geriaction: Provides information and support for all workers in the field through its newsletter and seminars.

Appendix C
Audiovisual Resources

Below are listed audiovisual resources relevant to aged care and a source list of suppliers. The films may also be available from local film libraries, and most will arrange interlibrary loan if a film is not available. Many charity and disability associations also have films and videos for hire, and are developing new material all the time. The relevant organisation should be approached wherever necessary. Many will only lend their material to members, but will often be willing to send out a representative with a film. Films can also be obtained through the libraries of colleges and universities, the Association of Occupational Therapists, and other professional associations in each State (see Appendix B for addresses).

Sources

Ask each organisation for the current list of their films and videos.

National

Australian Broadcasting Corpoation (ABC). Inquire through the ABC Film Library in each State

ACROD (*see under Ageing for the State Offices, Appendix A*)

State Film Centres in each capital

Victoria.
Tel area code (03)

Alzheimer Society of Victoria, 98 Riversdale Road, Hawthorn VIC 3122. Tel: 818 3022.

Arthritis Foundation Of Victoria, Yarra Boulevard, Kew VIC 3101. Tel: 862 2555.

Association for the Blind, 7 Main Street, Brighton VIC 3186. Tel: 598 8555.

Australian Film Institute, 49 Eastern Road, South Melbourne VIC 3205. Tel: 696 1844.

Carringbush Library, 415 Church Street, Richmond VIC 3121. Tel: 429 3644.

Early Planning for Retirement Association (EPRA), 459 Swanston Street, Melbourne VIC 3000. Tel: 663 3235.

Educational Media Australia Pty Ltd Film Producers (EMA), 7 Martin Street, South Melbourne VIC 3205. Tel: 699 7144.

Mayfield Centre (*see under Staff Development Centres, Appendix B*).

Queen Elizabeth Centre, 102 Ascot Street, Ballarat VIC 3205. Tel: (053) 321 811.

Royal Guide Dog Association, Private Mailbag 13, Kew VIC 3101. Tel: 860 4444.

State Film Centre, 17 St Andrews Place, East Melbourne VIC 3350. Tel: 651 1301.

Council On the Ageing (*see under Ageing, Appendix A*)

South Australia.
Tel area code (08)

South Australian Film Corporation, 113 Tapley Hill Road, Hendon SA 5014. Tel: 348 9300.

University of South Australia, Faculty of Health and Biomedical Sciences. School of Occupational Therapy, PO Box 2471, Adelaide SA 5000. North Terrace, Adelaide SA 5000. Tel: 302 2484.*

New South Wales.
Tel area code (02)

Cumberland College of Health Sciences, University of Sydney, PO Box 170, Lidcome NSW 2141. East Street, Lidcome NSW 2141. Tel: 646 6444.*

Queensland.
Tel area code (07)

University of Queensland, Department of Occupational Therapy, Therapies Building, St Lucia QLD 4072. Tel: 365 2652, 365 2820.*

Western Australia.
Tel area code (09)

Curtin University of Technology, Schools of Therapy, Selby Street, Shenton Park WA 6008. Tel: 381 0600.*

Audiovisual Resources

The following list indicates the range of material available. This material is compiled with the assistance of information from Barbara Davison of Lincoln Institute. Used with permission.

Key to type of A/V material: V = video   F = 16 mm film   K = kit   A/C = audio cassette   ST = slide tape.

Health Problems and Care

Incontinence	F	All Our Tomorrows	F
Explosions in the Mind (strokes)	V	Nell and Fred	F
ASTRA (on confusion)	F	Who Cares Anyway?	F
An Introduction to Residential Care (ACROD)	K	Nobody Ever Died of Old Age	F
		Ageing	F
An Inner Music — the Body Ear	A/C	Hattie	F
Not without Sight	F	The Facts are These: Three Score	
Stroke: How to Cope	V	Years and Ten	F
		Cemetery of the Elephant	F

Ageing

		Dear Theo	F
		Everybody Rides the Carousel	F
Really Good Friends (student tutorship program)	F/V	For Gentlemen Only	F
Transplant	F	Gerontology: Learning about Ageing	F

---

* Denotes the campuses where paramedical science courses are run. They will each have extensive libraries, including audiovisual material for loan for educational purposes. The libraries should also be able to direct inquirers to the suppliers of films they do not hold.

How We Adapt F
In Time F
The Last of Life F
A New Age for the Old F
Portraits of Ageing F
Priory: The Only Name I've Got F

Death and Bereavement

Death: Coping with Loss (US) F
Aspects of Bereavement F
Widowhood F
Dealing with Death A/C
Death and Dying A/C
To Die Today F

Nursing Homes

We are All Alone, My Dear F
Peege F
The Wild Goose F
Honey (pets in institutions) V

Housing

Beyond Shelter: the Problems of
  Housing the Elderly F

Older Women

The Invisible Woman F
Age Before Beauty F

Autonomy for the Aged

Mr B. Says No F
Do Do (autonomy for the aged) V
Mrs R. V

Leisure

Close Harmony (intergenerational
  music exchange) F

Reality Orientation

Reality Orientation Kit (6 parts;
  American Hospital Association;
  good on attitudes of staff) K, S/T
December Spring: 24-hour Reality
  Orientation F
A Time to Learn: Reality
  Orientation in a Nursing Home F
Return to Reality F
This Way to Reality S/T

Retirement

Work and Retirement (UK) F
A Time for Living F
The Big Day F
A Time to Look Forward (UK) F
The Challenging Years F
Retirement: Planning and
  Attitudes A/C
Twenty Years of Twilight A/C

Community Education

Care for the Elderly at Home
  (6 parts) V
a) Introduction by Geriatrician
b) Practical Nursing Management
c) Transfers, Mobility, Aids
d) Community Support Services
e) Recreation Ideas for the Depressed
  and Lonely
f) Coping with Grief and Stress
(Available through VAOT, Victorian
  Association of Occupational Therapy,
  Public Relations Officer.)

Films for Entertainment

Movielink Film Distributors: 8–10 River Street, Richmond VIC 3121. Tel: (03) 428 8088. Distributors of commercial feature-length movies, with a particularly good range of the old MGM greats. Their films are always in excellent condition and they also offer a courier service. Well worth it (see under Films in Chapter 4).

Videos from the EMA (Educational Media Australia)

Not Alone Anymore: Caring for
  Someone with Alzheimer's
  Disease V
Pills Unlimited V
Rose by Any Other Name V
Search for Intimacy: Love, Sex
  and Relationships in the Senior
  Years V
Second Debut V

Staying On: Living at Home Safely V
Dealing with Alzheimer's:
  A Common Approach to
  Communication V
Dealing with Alzheimer's: Facing
  Difficult Decisions V
Detecting Dementia V
Don't Take my Sunshine Away V
Living with Dying V
Molly and Max V

Appendix D
Serial Publications and Books

There are many publications available which provide continuing information about aged care. The following serials are held at the Council on the Ageing (Australia), Meriel Wilmot Library, 3rd floor, VACC House, 464 St Kilda Road, Melbourne VIC 3004. Tel: (03) 820 2655. Council on the Ageing (Australia) has written many reports and submissions relevant to ageing; a list can be obtained from their library.

Aboriginal Health Information Bulletin, [Biannual] Australian Institute of Health and Welfare, GPO Box 570, Canberra ACT 2601.

The Accreditor: Newsletter of the Australian Council on Healthcare Standards (ACHS), [3 per year] Australian Council on Healthcare Standards, 1st floor, 7–9a Joynton Ave, Zetland NSW 2017.

ACROD Newsletter, [9 per year] ACROD Ltd. Australia Council on Disability. PO Box 60, Curtin ACT 2605.

Action Network: Newsletter of the Australian Pensioners' and Superannuants' Federation Inc, [4–6 per year] Australian Pensioners' & Superannuants' Federation Inc, Suite 62, Level 6, 8–24 Kippax Street, Surry Hills 2010 NSW.

Activities Digest, PO Box 5227D, Newcastle West NSW 2302. *Activities Digest* is written to help organisers of activity programs for elderly or disabled people. Each issue has a variety of projects to help the organiser interest clients in maintaining health by taking part in simple keep-fit sessions, social events, crafts modified to suit special needs, and other planned activities. Most projects are quick to prepare and low in cost, and some programs can be used for fundraising events. Some topical news is included to help readers keep in touch with developments in aged care.

Age Exchange: Newsletter of the Intergenerational Activity Network, IAN, c/o Council on the Ageing (WA), 11 Freedman Rd, Mt Lawley WA 2133.

Age Pension News, [Irregular] Department of Social Security, PO Box 7788, Canberra ACT 2610.

Ageing Action, [Quarterly] Office of Ageing, Department of Family Services and Aboriginal and Islander Affairs, GPO Box 806, Brisbane QLD 4001.

Ageing and Society, [Quarterly] Cambridge University Press, The Edinburgh Building, Shaftesbury Rd, Cambridge CB2 2RU, U.K.

Ageing International, [Quarterly] International Federation on Ageing, 601 E St, NW, Washington DC 20049, USA.

Aging/MR IG Newsletter, [Quarterly] American Association of Mental Retardation and SIG on Mental

Retardation of the Gerontological Society of America.

Alzheimer's Newsletter, [Quarterly] Alzheimer's Association Western Australia. Corner Hammersley Rd and Thomas St, Subiaco WA 6008.

Alzheimer's Association South Australian Newsletter, Alzheimer's Association (SA) PO Box 202, Eastwood SA 5063.

ARPA News Victoria, [Monthly] Australian Retired Persons Association, 9th floor, 150 Queens Street, Melbourne VIC 3000.

Australian Association of Gerontology Newsletter, [Quarterly] Australian Association of Gerontology, Clunies Ross House, 191 Royal Pde, Parkville VIC 3052.

Australian Casemix Bulletin, [Irregular] Department of Health, Housing and Community Services, GPO Box 9848, Canberra ACT 2601.

Australian Disability Review, [Quarterly] AGPS for Disability Advisory Council of Australia, Canberra.

Australian Journal on Ageing, [Quarterly] Council on the Ageing (Australia). 3rd floor, 464 St Kilda Rd, Melbourne VIC 3004.

Australian Journal of Social Issues, [Quarterly] Australian Council of Social Service, PO Box E158, St James, Sydney NSW 2000.

Australian Senior Citizen, [Monthly] Australian Senior Citizen, PO Box 130, Wyong NSW 2259.

Australian Society for Geriatric Medicine Newsletter (previously Australian Geriatrics Society Newsletter), Australian Society for Geriatric Medicine, 145 Macquarie Street, Sydney NSW 2000.

The Bottom Line, [10 per year] Australian Pensioners' & Superannuants' Federation Inc, Suite 62, Level 6, 8–24 Kippax St, Surry Hills NSW 2010.

Brotherhood Action, [Quarterly] Brotherhood of St Laurence, 67 Brunswick St, Fitzroy VIC 3065.

Bulletin on Aging, [Biannual] United Nations Centre for Social Development and Humanitarian Affairs, International Centre, Box 500, A-1400, Vienna, Austria.

Carers Association of Australia Newsletter, Carers Association of Australia, PO Box 76, Lyons ACT 2606.

Carers Group Newsletter, [Monthly] Council on the Ageing (ACT) (sponsored).

The Comet: the Voice of Pensioners, [Monthly] Australian Pensioners' and Superannuants' League, Queensland Inc, PO Box 5141, West End QLD 4101.

Consumer Action, [Bimonthly] Australian Federation of Consumer Organisations, Level 1, 40 Mort Street, Braddon ACT 2601.

Consuming Interest, [Quarterly] Australian Consumers' Association, 57 Carrington Rd, Marrickville NSW 2204.

COTA (Australia) National News, [Quarterly] Council on the Ageing (Australia).

COTA News (NSW), [Quarterly] Council on the Ageing (NSW), 54 Argyle Place, Millers Point NSW 2000.

COTA News (TAS), [Quarterly] Council on the Ageing (TAS), 2 St Johns Avenue, New Town TAS 7008.

COTA News (QLD), Council on the Ageing (QLD) Inc, Sir Leslie Wilson Youth Centre, 2nd floor, Tenth Avenue, Windsor QLD 4030.

COTA News (SA), [Bimonthly] Council on the Ageing (SA), 45 Flinders St, Adelaide SA 5000.

COTA News (Vic), [Quarterly] Council on the Ageing (VIC), 126 Wellington Pde, Melbourne VIC 3002.

COTA Notes: Newsletter of the Council on the Ageing (ACT), Council on the Ageing (ACT), Hughes Community Centre, Hughes ACT 2605.

COTA (NT) Inc, Newsletter, 18 Bauhinia St, Nightcliff NT 0810.

Dementia Today, [Quarterly] Alzheimer's Association (Australia) Inc, PO Box 51, North Ryde NSW 2113.

Eagle: Exchange on Ageing, Law & Ethics, [Irregular] International Federation on Ageing, European Office, Astral House, 1268 London Rd, Norbury, London SW16 4EJ, U.K.

Eurolink Age Bulletin, [3 per year] Eurolink Age, 1268 London Rd, London SW16 4EJ, U.K.

Family Matters, [Quarterly] Australian Institute of Family Studies, 300 Queen St, Melbourne VIC 3000.

Fifty (50) Something, [Bimonthly] National Seniors Association, Sydney and Brisbane.

Geriaction, [Quarterly] Geriaction Inc, 4th floor, 282 Victoria Ave, Chatswood NSW 2067.

Geriaction Newsletter, Geriaction Victoria, PO Box 469, Hawthorn VIC 3122.

HACC Update: National Newsletter of the Home and Community Care Program, [Irregular] Department of Health, Housing and Community Services, GPO Box 9848, Canberra ACT 2601.

Health Forum, [Quarterly] Update to members (filed with Health Forum), Consumers' Health Forum of Australia, PO Box 52, Lyons ACT 2602.

Health Issues, [Quarterly] Health Issues Centre, 1st floor, 257 Collins St, Melbourne VIC 3000.

IFA Newsletter, Regional Newsletter on Ageing and Services for the Elderly, [Annual] International Federation on Ageing, Office of the Vice President for Asia, IFA, c/o Hong Kong Council of Social Service, GPO Box 474, Hong Kong.

Impact, [11 per year] ACOSS, PO Box 45, St James Square, Sydney NSW 2000.

The Independent Retiree, [Bimonthly] Marabridge Pty Ltd for Association of Independent Retirees, 33 Doggett Street, Newstead Qld 4006.

International Journal of Ageing and Human Development, [8 per year] Baywood Publishing Co, PO Box 337, Amityville NY 11701, USA.

Journals of Gerontology, [Bimonthly] Gerontological Society of America, 1275 K St NW, Suite 350, Washington DC 20005-4006, USA.

Leisure for Pleasure, Recreation for Older Adults SA Inc, 1 Sturt St, Adelaide SA 5000.

Link-Australia's Disability Magazine (incorporates Breakthrough), [Bimonthly] Disabled Peoples' International South Australian Branch, GPO Box 909, Adelaide SA 5000.

Links, [Quarterly] Consumers and General Practice Newsletter, Consumers' Health Forum, PO Box 52, Lyons ACT 2606.

Medicare Forum: A newsletter from the Health Insurance Commission, [Quarterly] Health Insurance Commission, PO Box 1001, Tuggeranong ACT 2901.

National Centre for Ageing and Sensory Loss Newsletter (NCASL), a division of the Association for the Blind Ltd, VIC, 7 Mair St, Brighton Beach VIC 3186.

Network News, [Biannual] a newsletter of the global link for midlife and older women, American Association of Retired Persons, in association with International Federation on Ageing, 601 E Street NW, Washington DC 20049, USA.

New Literature on Old Age: a guide to new publications, courses and conferences on ageing, [Bimonthly] Centre for Policy on Ageing Information Sevice, 25–31 Ironmonger Row, London ECV1 3QP, England.

New Times for Older Australians, [Quarterly] Department of Health, Housing and Community Services, GPO Box 9848, Canberra ACT 2601.

Pensioners' Voice, [11 per year] Combined Pensioners' and Superannuants' Association, Level 5, 405-411 Sussex St, Haymarket NSW 2000.

Residential Care News, [Irregular] AGPS for Department of Health, Housing and Community Services, Aged and Community Care Division.

Retirement Industry Journal, [Bimonthly] a journal for retirement villages, nursing homes, hospitals and health insurance industries. The Communication Organisation Pty Ltd, PO Box 513, Mudgeeraba QLD 4213.

Retirement Magazine, [Monthly] a monthly guide to planning and enjoying retirement. Chris Macleod and Mark Jamieson. PO Box 72, Caulfield South VIC 3162.

SHOP Newsletter, [Bimonthly] Self Help for Older People in Health Promotion Project, 2nd floor, Ross House, 247–251 Flinders Lane, Melbourne VIC 3000.

Social Security Journal, [Biannual] AGPS, GPO Box 84, Canberra ACT 2601.

Speaking Up, [Irregular] Older Persons' Action Centre, 256 Flinders St, Melbourne VIC 3000.

SPRC Newsletter, [Quarterly] Social Policy Research Centre, University of New South Wales, PO Box 1, Kensington NSW 2033.

Take Care, [Quarterly] Newsletter for non-profit providers of aged and disabled care, Aged Care Australia Inc, PO Box 303, Curtin ACT 2605.

Victorian Health Promotion Foundation Letter, [Quarterly] 1st floor, 333 Drummond St, Carlton South VIC 3053.

Welfare Rights Centre Newsletter, [Quarterly] Welfare Rights Centre, 4th floor, 245 Castlereagh St, Sydney NSW 2000.

Your Retirement: the Australian Retirement Guide, [Annual] National Publishing Group, 66 Foveaux St, Surry Hills NSW 2010.

Books

Various books are listed throughout the text which will provide useful reading. Council on the Ageing (Australia), Meriel Wilmot Library, has an extensive range of books specifically on aged care and policy. Topics covered include: Accommodation, Adult Education, Alzheimer's Disease, Bereavement, Community Care, Confusion, Day Care Centres, Death, Disabled, Education, Ethnic Communities, Family Welfare, Geriatric Medicine and Nursing, Homelessness, Immigration, Incontinence, Institutional Care, Leisure Activities, Mental Health, Nutrition, Psychological Ageing, Recreation, Rehabilitation, Terminal Care, Volunteer Services, Widowhood. The Library provides a useful resource centre and service.

Appendix E

Community Education Programs for Older Adults

The following list of resources has been drawn from the TAFE report: Beaton, H. (1986) *Learning in the Later Years.* TAFE, Victoria. It has been used with copyright permission from TAFE VIC. Copies of the report are available from TAFE or the Hawthorn Community Education Centre, 24 Wakefield Street, Hawthorn VIC 3122. Tel: (03) 819 8824, 819 5771.

Australian College for Seniors, Northfields Avenue, Wollongong NSW 2500. Tel: 008 025 473.

Australian College for Seniors, based at Riverina CAE. It provides low-cost residential programs, usually for a week, at universities, colleges of advanced education and other tertiary campuses around Australia. There are three recognisable divisions in a typical program:

(a) 'Knowledge and understanding' courses, such as psychology and environmental studies.

(b) 'Practical skills' courses such as painting, Tai Chi and computing.

(c) 'Business of living' courses such as nutrition, communication skills, ageing.

Carringbush Community Arts Program, Carringbush Regional Library, 415 Church Street, Richmond VIC 3121. Tel: (03) 429 3644.

Carrington Community Arts Program. One of the aims of this program in Melbourne is to teach theatre and film skills. The Tombola Players are older persons performing for the general public and people in nursing homes and kindergartens. In 1983/84 the group made an award-winning film called *Mr B. Says No*, about a man refusing to go into a nursing home.

SPAN, 298 Victoria Road, Thornbury VIC 3071. Tel: (03) 480 1364.

SPAN is a group of older people providing services to their local community. It runs a home repair service, a reading program with students from a local secondary school, an adult literacy program, social activities and lobbying of government departments. The program is run by volunteers, with a paid coordinator to provide continuity.

Universities of the Third Age (U3A), City Campus, Universities of the Third Age, c/-Council of Adult Education, 256 Flinders Street, Melbourne VIC 3000. Tel: (03) 652 0611.

Universities of the Third Age (U3A) Subjects of both academic and general interest are offered according to the resources of each campus. Tutors, students and organisers are all voluntary.

Over 60s Radio- 5UV Over 60s Radio 5UV, 228 North Terrace, Adelaide SA 5000. Tel: (08) 303 5000.

Over 60s Radio — 5UV is an educational radio station which began in 1979. It broadcasts from the University of Adelaide, from 2.30–5 pm each weekday. Volunteers prepare and present programs to an estimated audience of 50,000.

Older Persons Action Centre, c/- Council of Adult Education, 256 Flinders Street, Melbourne VIC 3000. Tel: (03) 652 0611.

Older Persons Action Centre (OPAC) is a group of older persons which seeks to have direct access to policy-makers at all levels of government. It is represented on Senior Citizens Week Advisory Committee, the Home and Community Care (HACC) Consultative Committee, the Health Issues Centre (HIC) Management Committee, and others. OPAC is also interested in self-education and often has speakers and workshops.

'Mind and Matter' kit for health programs, Health Promotion services, 189 Royal Street, West Perth WA 6005. Tel: (09) 222 4222.

'Mind and Matter' kit for health programs is designed for use by older people running programs. Topics include self-care, heart, keeping fit, being assertive, safety at home.

Learning for the Less Mobile (LLM), Hawthorn Community Education Centre, 24 Wakefield Street, Hawthorn VIC 3122. Tel: (03) 819 8824.

Learning for the Less Mobile (LLM). Discussion groups and film outings with older people from local nursing homes and hostels, using multipurpose taxis for transport.

Correspondence Courses for Housebound People Hawthorn Community Education Centre, Wakefield Street Hawthorn VIC 3122. Tel: (03) 819 8824.

Appendix F

Song Titles and Music

Song titles by theme: Compiled by Betty Stinson.

The following lists of song titles are grouped together for use in quizzes.

Home

My Old Kentucky Home
Take Me Home Again, Kathleen
Show Me the Way to go Home
Home on the Range

Little Grey Home in the West
Home Sweet Home
Green, Green Grass of Home
Take Me Home, Country Road

Colours

Blue Skies
Blue Moon
Blue Room
Bluebirds over the White Cliffs of
   Dover
Blue Danube
Lavender Blue
Green, Green Grass of Home
Wearing of the Green
My Blue Heaven
Bluebird of Happiness
Red Sails in the Sunset
Red River Valley

Red, Red Robin
Look for the Silver Lining
Yellow Submarine
Yellow Rose of Texas
Little Yellow Bird
Tie a Yellow Ribbon
Lemon Tree
White Christmas
Little White Cloud that Cried
White Magnolia Tree
Old Black Joe
Ten Green Bottles

First name

Charmaine
Dianne
Alice' Blue Gown
Wild about Harry
Sweet Caroline
Margie
Lilli Marlene
Heather on the Hill
Annie Laurie
Sally
Rose Marie
Waltzing Matilda

Kathleen
Champagne Charlie
Danny Boy
My Bonnie
Charlie My Boy
K-K-Katy
Sweet Lorraine
My Gal Sal
Wait till the Sun Shines, Nelly
Ida, Sweet as Apple Cider
Mona Lisa
Tammy

Goodnight, Irene
Pedro the Fisherman
Frankie and Johnny
Alexander's Ragtime Band
Daisy
Lily of Laguna
June is Busting Out all Over
Robert E. Lee
Rosie O'Grady
Nelly Kelly
Peggy O'Neil

Old Black Joe
O Johnnie
Billy Boy
Bill Bailey
If You Knew Suzie
Laura
Louise
Mary's a Grand Old Name
Rosalie
Georgie Girl
Abie my Boy

Flowers

Heather on the Hill
Lavender Blue
When You Wore a Tulip
Tulip From Amsterdam
Tiptoe through the Tulips
Daisy
Sweet Violets
Apple Blossom Time
We'll Gather Lilacs
Lily of Laguna
Bluebells of Scotland
Eidelweiss

Rose Marie
Moonlight and Roses
One Dozen Roses
Rose of Tralee
Roses of Picardy
Forget-me-not Lane
Mexicali Rose
Little Petunia in an Onion Patch
Honeysuckle Rose
Secondhand Rose
Last Rose of Summer
My Love is like a Red, Red Rose

Cities

Beautiful, Beautiful Copenhagen
Foggy Day in London Town
Road to Gundagai
Goodbye, Melbourne Town
In Dublin's Fair City

Tipperary
I Love Paris
I Belong to Glasgow
San Fransisco, Open Your Golden
    Gate

Birds

A Nightingale Sang in Berkeley
    Square
Red, Red Robin
Bye, Bye, Blackbird
Only a Bird in a Gilded Cage
Listen to the Mockingbird

When the Swallows Come Back
Bluebirds over the White Cliffs of
    Dover
Bluebird of Happiness
Skylark

Seasons and weather

Younger than Springtime
Springtime in the Rockies
Lazy, Hazy, Crazy Days of Summer
Summertime
Good old Summertime
September in the Rain
June is Busting Out all Over
Apple Blossom Time

Autumn Leaves
Let it Snow
Stormy Weather
Singin' in the Rain
June in January
Harvest Moon
A Foggy Day
Umbrella Man

I'll Remember April
April Showers
April in Paris

Sunny Side of the Street
Pennies from Heaven
The Sun has got His Hat On

Times of day

Three o'clock in the Morning
Good Morning
Red Sails in the Sunset
Night and Day
Goodnight, Sweetheart
Blues in the Night
Grand Night for Singing
Meet Me in Dreamland

Oh, What a Beautiful Morning
Sunrise Serenade
Moonglow
The Chapel in the Moonlight
Paper Moon
Blue Moon
Light of the Silvery Moon

Songs beginning with 'when'

The Swallows Come Back
Irish Eyes are Smiling
I Grow Too Old to Dream
You and I Were Young
The Blue of the Night
I'm Cleaning Windows

I'm 64
Your Hair has Turned to Silver
You Wish upon a Star
Whip o'Wills Call
The Red, Red Robin

Songs which begin with 'who'

Wants to be a Millionaire
Sorry Now

Stole my Heart Away

Songs which begin with 'if'

I Ruled the World
I had a Talking Picture of You
You Knew Suzie
I had My Life to Live Over

If These Lips Could Only Talk
My Friends Could See Me Now
You Were the Only Girl in the World

Father's Day

Oh, My Papa
My Grandfather's Clock

Daddy Wouldn't Buy Me a Bow-wow

Bastille Day

The Last Time I Saw Paris
Darling, Je Vous Aime Beaucoup
Sur le Pont

Mademoiselle from Armentiers
Gigi

Show time

Old Macdonald had a Farm
Swinging on a Star

Old Grey Mare
How Much is that Doggie in the
Window

Melbourne Cup

Camptown Ladies

Beedlehorn

Australia Day

Waltzing Matilda
Advance Australia Fair
Botany Bay
Goodbye, Melbourne Town
Road to Gundagai
Dog Sits on the Tuckerbox

I'm Going Back Again to Yarrawonga
Skippy
Click, Go the Shears
Kookaburra Sits in the Old Gum Tree
Tie me Kangaroo Down, Sport
Six White Boomers
Wild Colonial Boy

St Valentine's Day

My Funny Valentine
I Love you Truly
I'll be your Sweetheart
It's a Sin to Tell a Lie
Always
Sweetheart, Sweetheart, Sweetheart

My Hero
Love's Old Sweet Song
One Day When We Were Young
Anniversary Waltz
Goodnight, Sweetheart
Girls were Made to Love and Kiss

Moomba

The More We are Together

The Carnival is Over

Anzac Day

Bless 'em All
We'll Meet Again
Pack Up Your Troubles
Tipperary
Keep the Home Fires Burning

Lilli Marlene
White Cliffs of Dover
Roses of Picardy
Mademoiselle from Armentiers

Empire Day

Rule Britannia
There'll Always be an England

English Country Garden
Old Father Thames

Mother's Day

Mother Macree
Did Your Mother Come from Ireland
Little Old Lady Passing By
Ma, He's Making Eyes at Me

M-O-T-H-E-R
Mama
Song My Mother Taught Me
The Silver in My Mother's Hair

St Patrick's Day

Wearing the Green
Great Day for the Irish
Mountains of Mourne
Rose of Tralee
Where the River Shannon Flows
Galway Bay
Danny Boy
Mother Macree
I'll Take You Home Again, Kathleen
Phil the Fluter's Ball

Peggy O'Neil
Paddy McGinty's Goat
Harrigan
If You're Irish, Come into the
    Parlour
Kathleen Mavourneen
Mollie Malone
Nellie Kelly
Come Back to Erin
Irish Lullaby

Macushla   Irish Eyes are Smiling
Macnamara's Band

Songs from different eras: Compiled by Mary Ward.

These lists are useful to ensure that the music which is selected will be appropriate to the age of the people in the group.

Songs of the twenties (the jazz age; a gaudy, bawdy, totally desperate decade; the Charleston to the Crash)

Ain't Misbehaving
Ain't She Sweet
Among My Souvenirs
Baby Face
Charmaine
Dinah
Don't Bring Lulu
Five Foot Two, Eyes of Blue
Girl of My Dreams
I can't Give You Anything but Love
I'll be with You in Apple Blossom Time
I'm just Wild about Harry

It had to be You
Last Night on the Back Porch
Manhattan
My Blue Heaven
Ramona
Secondhand Rose
Side by Side
Singin' in the Rain
That's My Weakness Now
Toot Toot Tootsie
When You're Smiling
Who's Sorry Now
You were Meant for Me

Songs of the thirties (the Depression decade, dole queues and tough times; murmurs of war)

A Tisket a Tasket
Auf Wiedersehen, My Dear
Between the Devil and the Deep Blue Sea
Blue Moon
Careless Love
Harbour Lights
Have You Ever been Lonely
Ida, Sweet as Apple Cider
I Only have Eyes for You

It Happened in Monterey
Lady of Spain
Lazy Bones
Lullaby of Broadway
On the Sunny Side of the Street
Red Sails in the Sunset
So Deep is the Night
Stardust
Stormy Weather

Songs of the forties (the Second World War)

Almost like Being in Love
A Nightingale sang in Berkeley Square
Chattanooga Choo Choo
Coming in on a Wing and a Prayer
Deep in the Heart of Texas
Elmer's Tune
Fascination
Granada
Heart of My Heart

Moonlight Serenade
My Guy's Come Back
My Heart and I
Now is the Hour
Old Shep
Paper Doll
Red Roses for a Blue Lady
The Gypsy
White Cliffs of Dover
You are My Sunshine

Jealousy
Laura
Lazy River
Lilli Marlene

You Belong to My Heart
You're Nobody 'til Somebody Loves
  You
Yours

Songs of the fifties (the aftermath of the war; a decade of progress; the age of the crooner and the birth of rock 'n' roll)

All the Way
An Affair to Remember
Answer Me
Cara Mia
Eternally
Fly Me to the Moon
From a Jack to a King
Green Door
High Noon
Hi-Lili, Hi Lo
If I had a Hammer
Jailhouse Rock
Kisses Sweeter than Wine
Love is a Many Splendoured Thing

Catch a Falling Star
C'est Si Bon
Cry
Ebb Tide
Love Me Tender
Milord
Oh, My Papa
Peggy Sue
Secret Love
The Tender Trap
Three Coins in a Fountain
Too Young
Volare

Music for opening a session

Alexander's Ragtime Band
Bingo
Consider Yourself at Home
Do Re Me
Funiculi Funicula

Getting to Know You
Happy Days are Here Again
The Happy Wanderer
The More We are Together
Seventy-Six Trombones

Music for closing a session

After the Ball is Over
Alohe Oe
Always
Auld Lang Syne
Goodnight, Irene
Goodnight, Sweetheart

I Could have Danced all Night
I'll See You Again
So Long, It's been Good to Know
  You
Show Me the Way to Go Home

Hits of the war years

Knees up, Mother Brown
When the Lights Go Off All Over the
  World
It's a Long Way to Tipperary
Pack up Your Troubles in Your Old
  Kit Bag
Nursie Nursie
We're Going to Hang out the Washing
  on the Siegfried Line
Run Rabbit Run

Wish Me Luck as You Wave Me
  Goodbye
We'll Meet Again
Colonel Bogey
The White Cliffs of Dover
Lilli Marlene
Over There
The Marines Hymn
Now is the Hour
Round Off

Kiss Me Goodnight, Sergeant Major
It's a Lovely Day Tomorrow
In the Quartermaster's Store
Keep the Home Fires Burning
Mademoiselle from Armentieres
Take Me Back to Dear Old Blighty
Beer Barrel Polka
Till the Lights of London Shine
Again

The Caissons go Rollin' Along
US Airforce March
Moonlight Serenade
American Patrol
St Louis Blues March
Bless 'em All
Waltzing Matilda

Popular songs

After the Ball
Always
Amazing Grace
Auf Wiedersehen, Sweetheart
Are You Lonesome Tonight
Babyface
The Band Played On
Barbara Allen
The Beer Barrel Polka
Bendemeer's Stream
A Bird in a Gilded Cage
Blue Moon
Blue-Tailed Fly
Born Free
Botany Bay
Breezin' Along with the Breeze
Bye, Bye, Blackbird
Bye Bye Blues
By the Light of the Silvery Moon
Cecilia
Carolina in the Morning
Catch a Falling Star
Charmaine
Cindy
Clementine
Click, Go the Shears
Cockles and Mussels
Cruising Down by the River
Daisy
Dance with a Dolly
Danny Boy
Don't Bring Lulu
Down by the Old Mill Stream
Down By the Riverside
Dream
Drunken Sailor
Edelweiss
English Country Garden
Forever and Ever
Four-Leaf Clover

Heart of My Heart
Glory of Love
Grandfather's Clock
Gypsy Rover
Happy Wanderer
Have You Ever Been Lonely
Hello, Hello, Who's Your Lady
Friend
Hello, My Baby
Home on the Range
Hush, Little Baby
I Belong to Glasgow
I Dream of Jeannie
I'd Like to Teach the World to Sing
I'm an Old Cowhand
I do Like to be Beside the Seaside
If You Knew Susie
If You were the Only Girl in the
World
I Know Where I'm Going
I'll be with You in Apple Blossom
Time
I'll String Along with You
I Love a Lassie
I Love You Truly
I'm Always Chasing Rainbows
I'm Henry the VIII, I am
In the Chapel in the Moonlight
Irene, Goodnight
The Isle of Innisfree
Istanbul
It Had to Be You
It's a Great Day for the Irish
It's a Long Way to Tipperary
It's been a Long, Long Time
I've got a Lovely Bunch of Coconuts
I Want a Girl
I Wonder Who's Kissing Her Now
Jamaican Farewell
Knees up, Mother Brown

Lavender Blue
Let Me Call You Sweetheart
Lilli Marlene
Lily of Laguna
Little White Duck
Little Yellow Bird
Love is Blue
Love Letters in the Sand
Loch Lomond
Lullaby of Broadway
Loveliest Night of the Year
Mademoiselle of Armentieres
Mairzy Doats (Mares eat Oats)
Makin' Whoopee
Marie
Mary's a Grand Old Name
Mary Lou
Maybe It's Because I'm a Londoner
Me and My Shadow
Memories
Michael, Row the Boat Ashore
Moonlight Bay
Morning has Broken
My Bonnie is over the Ocean
My Blue Heaven
Nelly Kelly, I Love You
A Nice Cup of Tea
Now is the Hour
Oh Johnny, Oh Johnny, Oh
Oh, My Papa
Oh, Susanna
Old Folks at Home
On the Sunny Side of the Street
Over the Rainbow
Pack up Your Troubles in Your Old
　Kit Bag
Paper Doll
Peg o' My Heart
Pretty Baby
Que ser'a, ser'a
Red Roses for a Blue Lady
Riddle Song
Roamin' in the Gloamin'
The Rose of Tralee
Row Row Row
Rudolph, the Red-nosed Reindeer
Sail along Silvery Moon
Sioux City Sue
Sentimental Journey
She'll be Coming Round the
　Mountain
Shine on Harvest Moon

Side by Side
So Long, It's been Good to Know You
Sonny Boy
Singin' in the Rain
Skye Boat Song
A Star Fell from Heaven
Streets of Laredo
Swanee
Sweet Georgia Brown
Sweet Rosie O'Grady
Take Me Out to the Ball Game
That Lucky Old Sun
That's an Irish Lullaby
There is a Tavern in the Town
There's a Rainbow Round My
　Shoulder
They Didn't Believe Me
Tie Me Kangaroo Down
Till We Meet Again
Tiptoe through the Tulips
Too Young
Two Little Girls in Blue
Unicorn
What do You Want to Make Those
　Eyes at Me for?
Walking My Baby Back Home
When I Grow too Old to Dream
When I'm 64
When Irish Eyes are Smiling
Where Have All the Flowers Gone
Where the Blue of the Night
When the Red, Red Robin
When You're Smiling
Whispering
Who's Sorry Now
The White Cliffs of Dover
Yes Sir, That's My Baby
You are My Sunshine
You Made Me Love You

Silent Night
The First Noel
Mary's Boy Child
I Saw Three Ships
Good King Wenceslas
O Come, All ye Faithful
Jingle Bells
Hark, the Herald Angels Sing
Angels We have Heard on High
We Three Kings of Orient Are
O Faithful Pine (Tannenbaum)
Away in a Manger (three verses)

Action songs

John Brown's Baby (to the tune of 'John Brown's Body')
John Brown's baby has a cold upon its chest, (repeat three times)
And they rubbed it with camphorated oil.
(Actions: pointing to self, rock baby, sniff or blow nose, rub chest)
Chorus
Glory, glory, Hallelujah
(repeat three times, conducting with hands)
And they rubbed it with camphorated oil.

Head, Shoulders, Knees and Toes[1] (to the tune of 'There is a Tavern in the Town')
Head, shoulders, knees and toes, knees and toes.
(repeat, and)
Eyes and ears and nose,
Head, shoulders, knees and toes, knees and toes.

Hokey Pokey: Those who cannot stand, can clap their hands, or roll their hands, instead of standing and turning around.

Hands and Knees and Boomps a Daisy: Actions follow words of song.

He's Got the Whole World in His Hands: Actions follow words of song.

Heel and Toe Polka: Can be done sitting in chair.

Rheumatism (to the tune of Frere Jacques; a round; seated on a chair)
Rheumatism, rheumatism,
Oh! the pain, Oh! the pain, (face grimace)
Up and down the system, (stand up and down from the chair)
Up and down the system,
When it rains, when it rains. (rain with finger movements)

This round can be a lot of fun, as people are popping up and down at different times.

Reference

1. BRIGHT, Ruth. *Music in Geriatric Care*. Angus and Robertson, Sydney, 1972.

Index

CPSIA information can be obtained
at www.ICGtesting.com
Printed in the USA
LVOW13s0008270617
539398LV00005BA/629/P

9 781542 466165